When, Not If

Not a diary, not a journal,
just a conversation with myself.

By
Susan Scouller

THE STORY OF HER JOURNEY THROUGH
TREATMENT FOR BREAST CANCER

The proceeds from the sale of this book will be donated
to support research into finding a cure for Breast Cancer,
in particular the Candles charity.

First Published in Great Britain in 2005
by **TUCANN***books*
Text © Malcolm Scouller
All rights reserved
Design © **TUCANN***design&print*

ISBN N° 1 873257 56 2

Published by TUCANN*books*,
19 High Street, Heighington, Lincoln LN4 1RG
Tel & Fax: 01522 790009
www.tucann.co.uk

PREFACE

This story was written by my wife days or weeks after the events and is not a complete record of our last eighteen months together. There were a few months in the summer of 2003, when we thought she had beaten the cancer and we looked forward to many years together, especially as she appeared fit and well enough to visit the gym. She started these writings after it was suggested to her "why not write a book". I don't think she ever intended to publish it; however I feel the story should be told, warts and all. The process of typing it into the computer helped me understand what she had gone through, because although I had read bits of it, it only makes sense when it is read as a whole.

I would like to thank all Sue's friends who helped her through her illness, both the good times and the bad times. I would also like to thank all the medical staff who dealt with us during those difficult times.

I did remark to Sue one day, "that you have to be fit to be ill", while we waited for one of her many appointments. Some people manage to carry on working and running a family, while undergoing treatment. Luckily for us, Sue was retired and I was made redundant a year before she died, which meant we had much more time together. I however, salute all those who face cancer and whatever the outcome, the road must be very lonely at times, however many people are there to support you.

INTRODUCTION

I met Sue in 1978, when I joined The Royal Observer Corps; just by chance I went along on a Tuesday evening in response to a Recruitment leaflet delivered to my house. At first I did not take much notice of Sue, she I understand thought I looked unhappy and must be married with lots of children, I paid more attention to some of the new female recruits. Sue who lived in Branston, was a special schools teacher and really enjoyed her work with the children at Queen's Park.

We first went out together in the summer of 1979, got engaged at Christmas and were married the following summer on 26th July 1980.

PART 1.

IF

If They think I've gone potty,
And I'm sitting on my botty,
They are wrong!

If They think po-si-tive thought,
A bit of string the thing,
Then they are wrong!

If They think, I'll turn to drink,
And vote for Tony Blair,
They are wrong!

If I can keep my nerve and will,
I'll save the NHS a bill,
And - which is more - - -
I'll be right!

Dedicated to my in/out-laws, with apologies and acknowledgement to Rudyard Kipling.

S.S 11/2002

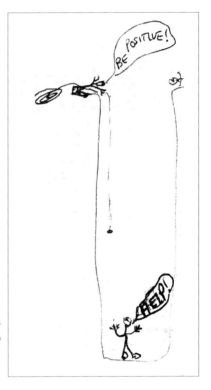

"The best way out is always through"

Robert Frost 1874-1963 'A servant to servants' (1914)

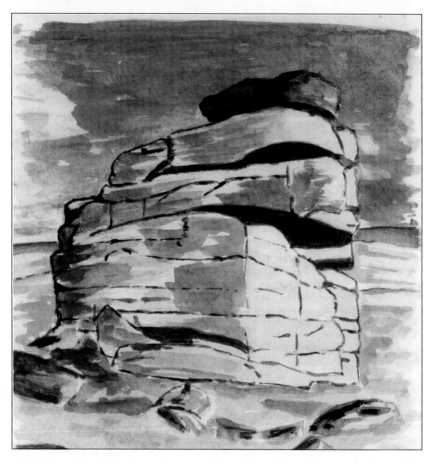

WHEN

When! Not if, they shouted sharply in my ear.

I looked at them, the oncologist and Macmillan nurse, both waiting for my reaction. My eyes, unfocused, my brain went straight into survival mode.

I had just had my Breast Cancer diagnosis confirmed. Would I like more information about chemotherapy and treatment? Yes, I was treatable; they needed more tests to see where it had spread to, liver, bones or brain. Yes I agreed they needed to know for their treatment preparation. No, I would not mind losing my hair, I would agree to anything they said, after all, I had no choice. I was going to be their best patient. I didn't want to be cast into the 'waste of money' box. I even remembered my manners and thanked them for their efforts on my behalf.

I went home on auto pilot, husband by my side, surprised that he had coped so well so far. He being, the highly strung and not used to having the medical thunder stolen from him.

I was feeling pretty sore from the biopsy tests. Never had I had so much attention in my life, even if it did consist of firing an aspiration gun at my breast, more alarming than painful. Never had so many men peer at and stroked my breast albeit with gel and sensors. Never had I met with so many kind, caring people, total strangers. Never have I been offered so many cups of tea.

Being in shock and feeling ill did have its compensations. X-ray, blood tests, ECG were completed in record time. One look at my ghastly pale face and they got rid of me as quickly as possible. Didn't want me to die on their patch!

Go home and wait for chemotherapy counselling and test results. Oh! Those test results, will they change their minds? The NHS needs money, the news that night was full of it.

No, escape in sleep, how can you sleep with legs shaking uncontrollably, so much that Malcolm nearly rattled out of bed.

No tears, surprised at that, speechless when I tried to tell my mother, opened my mouth, not a word would come out.

Friends, flew to my side, phone calls, offers of practical help, moral support, even my sister turned to, glad of a reason to break her lifelong "huff" with me, so long we had forgotten how it started.

Not so brave as I thought I could be. Bone scan result showed a problem with my bones, more X-rays needed. One look at the skeleton scan and I gave up the ghost.

· · · · · ·

HAIR TODAY, GONE TOMORROW

They knew I'd get a wig and I did,
They knew what I'd do.

I thought I wasn't vain,
A "wig!" are you insane.

They knew what I' do,
They knew I'd get a wig and I did.
"Bother"

S. Scouller 12/02

· · · · · ·

Veronica, my self appointed fashion adviser came along for my wig fitting. I took one look at the wigs lined up on the trolley and decided they looked like curled up cats and said I hoped they had been fed. (Why can't I stop making flippant remarks?)

The wig lady expert had chosen two for me. Feeling like Goldilocks, I said the first one was too brown, the second too grey. Wig lady expert started to look desperate and remembered a rejected moggie stuffed at the back of the trolley. Relief all round, mongrel moggie was just right, even down to the salt and pepper, wind blown effect.

Showed off my wig to startled husband who noticed it wasn't as dark brown as my own hair. If only he knew how difficult it had been to choose, he wouldn't have been so pedantic. Tempted to say he could borrow it for his bald head.

Veronica took me for a coffee to celebrate success of a difficult mission. We entertained each other with stories, mine of Malcolm trying to be the perfect husband and my hospital experiences. So much laughing could almost forget I had cancer at all. Decided that was exactly what I needed.

Veronica said I should write it all in a book, second person to say that, perhaps I will. Thanked God again for such good, kind friends.

My stubbornness to keep my hair for at least the second chemotherapy treatment backfired. Dr. E. was disappointed to see it was still there. I had to explain it had mostly fallen out a week ago and was only still there because I had left it alone. I then came unstuck with my choice of jumper (polo neck). Dr. E. sorted that out with great patience and tact and did some checking of progress.

I had only dared to feel one lump for size three weeks into the treatment, I thought it was smaller but braced myself for wishful thinking. Dr. E. seemed pleased and thought it was smaller. I wanted to ask five thousand questions including if this was normal progress or good progress in comparison with the average person. Thought I better not, just be satisfied with *SMALLER*.

Went home and combed out all of the remaining hair, fascinated by all the lumps and bumps on my scalp and the size of my head.

Very pleased that the ultrasound of my abdomen had been reported clear. Can't quite believe it, tempted to go through it bit by bit, just to be sure, but did not want to spoil the good news effect. Brain still in hiding, glad of the rest.

· · · · · ·

CHEMO' CLUB

GOOD AND CLEAR

If all the good people were clever,
And all clever people were good,
The world would be nicer than ever
We thought that it possibly could.

But somehow tis seldom or never,
The two hit it off as they should,
The good are so harsh to the clever,
The clever, so rude to the good!

> So friends, let it be our endeavour
> To make each by each understood,
> For few can be good, like the clever,
> Or clever, so well as the good.

Elizabeth Wordsworth 1840-1932

• • • • • •

15/12/02

Very concerned about the chemotherapy, didn't want to let my side down by not taking the session well. Very glad to be on a different day to Breast Cancer people. Like being with a mixture of men and old folk.

Ward looked more like a hotel or airport lounge, staff very friendly. Nurses make a big effort to help me and the whole thing went very well. The drugs went surging round my face and arms, everywhere. Must learn to let people get on with their job and stop checking. Frantic to get pill instruction correct, put it all in writing.

Feeling far too happy and relaxed for my own good must be going potty. Very glad to hand over responsibility for my medical welfare to people who have persuaded me (biggest doubting Thomas ever, where medics are concerned) that they know what they are doing.

Full of pills and notice a distinct stroppiness. "Banned" from Sainsbury's for rude comments at the check out. "Banned" from X-ray department for lack of patience. Gave a white van a run for its money up Canwick Hill. I'm turning into a monster. Husband being gingered up. Instructed not to climb ladders or mend anything, very unfair to him.

Beth, my Macmillan nurse rang to see how I am doing, very pleased with myself.

Off the hospital pills and flat on my face. Sick all night, days five, six and seven. Very close to giving up. How on earth am I going to manage this for three weeks? Never felt so ill, on my knees and not praying, except to shoot off some rapid arrow prayers, very short and to the point "HELP".

Dr. S. arrives and prescribes pills, take one and I am completely paralysed, can't possibly be sick, can't possibly move, not looking forward to this next time. Too exhausted to care. Malcolm, not letting me give up.

Surface at weekend, feel better, even with all the drugs going round, must have been feeling aweful before and refused to notice. Memo to body: - "I apologise for not listening to you."

Malcolm is in charge of cooking, doing wonders with soup, jelly, fish, mashed potato, loves being praised for efforts, decides he didn't like his jumper after all, too small from putting it in the washer. Decides easier to throw trousers away than wash them, spilt mercury on them after breaking weather thermometer. Has learnt that shopping trolleys are chained up, food doesn't stay in the fridge and shops are full of women cooing over babies.

Still worried that I'm not worried, must check with Beth, wonder when the fatigue and depression will start. Should be out of my mind with worry, perhaps this is normal, a defence mechanism. How can I be happy? Can only think it is all the new and unexpected realisation of how good everyone is when given a chance. Very proud of my friends who have busily knitted a safety net under and around me. Feel I didn't deserve any of it.

"NEVER ARGUE WITH A WOMAN ON PILLS."

Garage mechanic.

• • • • • •

ADVICE

"I always pass on good advice,
It's the only thing to do with it
It's never any use to oneself."

Oscar Wilde 1854-1900

OMENS
GOOD ONLY.

1) Saw complete double rainbow outside our house just after bad news. Last time I saw one of these was when my early retirement came through!

2) Garage serviced my car on time and charged less than the price quoted.

3) Prayer front well covered from Mormons, Happy Clappy, non-conformists, Church of England, candles lit in St. Hughs R.C, St. Peter and Pauls R.C and the cathedral no less! If that's not good, I don't know what is!!

4) Notice only one thing about Beth, she has brown eyes. My father had brown eyes.

5) Attended mobile screening unit two weeks before thyroid operation, narrow squeak.

6) Won fifty pounds on the Premium Bonds.

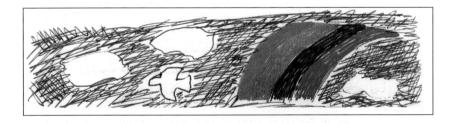

SELF PITY

I never saw a wild thing sorry for itself.
A small bird will drop frozen dead from a bough
Without ever having felt sorry for itself.

D.H Lawrence

Beth is my Macmillan nurse, yes, I know 'share' and quite right too, but Beth is my Macmillan nurse. A good start, the name pronunciation test went well, with a good stab at it. Thank goodness, no theoretical waffle, just brisk efficiency, fielded every question, and didn't take advantage of my vulnerability. Didn't seem to mind how many times she had to repeat answers to the simplest of questions. Took control, didn't mind being tested, didn't let me get out of control. Knew I wasn't going to be fobbed off with "be positive" came up with a logical answer to why I should be treated. Thank goodness she wasn't too "lovey dovey", I would have given in then. Every suggestion tried and proved to work. Maybe if Beth thinks I've got a chance and I can rely on Beth, maybe I have got a chance. Don't want to let Beth's faith in my getting better, down. Want to do well. Beth's bank of respect increasing, feeling very lucky to have a Beth.

I realise after 33 years of working with children in special schools, handicapped and behaviour problems, I am being given a hefty dose of my own medicine. All the things I said and did coming back to me, propping up parents, demoralised, aggressive, humiliated, vulnerable, argumentative, denying.

In need of good old fashioned common-sense, practical help and a sense of purpose.

Need to know if Beth has a sense of humour, much too professional to have one yet, decide to take a risk and show Beth my poem and burbling's.

MY ONCOLOGIST

"I left the room with silent dignity, but caught my foot in the mat." *

The diary of a nobody - Grossmith (1894)

* ME

I've learnt a new word, oncologist. Dr. E. has become transposed in my mind as Dr. Bad News. Grossly unfair, she only wanted to do the decent thing and give me the test results herself. Results, I had pestered to know I gave the impression I could take on the chin.

Learning quickly the rules of this horrid new game. No bad news over the phone, only the truth given. Trouble is patient in danger of being killed by all the truth.

How could I have argued and challenged the facts, risked alienating the very person trying to help me. How will I face another consultation again? Gave in to self-pity, hate myself. Give in and insist on only Good News, if any, at next day's appointment. Feel a wimp. Brain decides to veto any more reality. Glad brain has taken over, but I know I must face it sometime.

Not expecting to be called into consulting room before second chemotherapy treatment. Panic stations, insist good friend Sue comes with me and sits in. Dr. E. sorts out the sickness and pills, very pleased about this. Wants to check progress, didn't give much away except said it was smaller. Decide to save up questions for next consultation, work out one third should have gone, but maybe it doesn't work like that. Need to know about the blood, tumour markers, must understand every little bit.

I'm sorry I can't hear,
I've a suppository in my ear!

14

Can't wait to report back to Mum and Malcolm and sister. Sue, a brick, sat through the chemo' and provided me with diversion with the Ingham ward Christmas Quiz. Have great fun filling in patient questionnaire, discover whole room listening in and awaiting my answer to the one about sex. Ring both answers, must be joking, holding hands is about all either of us is capable of, very happy with new improved husband.

Surprised how competitive I am about the Christmas Quiz and keen to fill it in. Sainsbury's Customer Care provides answer to one about Snow White's Seven Dwarfs. Supervisor provides answer to another one. Completely forgot I have my wig on, no one seems to notice, more interested in the quiz, than my hair. Make mental note not to walk under any low decorations and get taffled up. Happiness thermometer going up again.

GOALS

1) I've bought a Christmas pudding and I hate waste.

2) Determined to see and hear new bells at Potterhanworth. Maybe I will be able to ring one of the light ones. Christopher has said I am to be in the team to ring the first quarter peal, to celebrate new bells, desperately want to join in celebrations. Have enjoyed supporting their fund raising efforts and admire Christopher's interest and dedication for a young teenager. Must learn methods and keep in practise.

3) Plenty of time to practise my painting, Malcolm very keen to encourage me, must try something new and bold.

4) Finish wild life pond.

5) Plant more trees at bottom of garden.

6) Design conservatory layout (Malcolm said)

7) Sit still through chemotherapy, so bleeper doesn't sound.

8) Visit New Zealand. (Check climate first)

9) Read all my books!

10) Get my ears pierced and only ears!

11) Survive to annoy my in-laws.

12) Learn to spell. Learn to do fractions.

THE OUT-LAWS

"We are all in the gutter, but some of us are looking at the stars"

Oscar Wilde 1854-1900

Malcolm reports news of my Breast Cancer to father during one of his regular phone calls. His father sent his best wishes, not love note, and said if I wished to cry on his shoulder I could, but not now, there was a programme on the TV he wanted to watch.

Malcolm very tired after looking after me during three nights of sickness, so I sent him to bed, he is exhausted, very worried and shocked. I surfaced and enjoyed watching programme about the religious architectural significance of the building of Durham Cathedral, concentrated and learnt quite a lot. So in happy mood when father-in-law rings. He enquires where Malcolm is and wants to speak to him, I explain why not, I'm not going to wake him, but demands he rings next night. So far no enquiry as to how I am, wonder how long it will be before he does; three quarters of the way through the call he asks about me, you would think I have chickenpox!

This year Malcolm and I have been up to Ullapool (500 miles) three times, each time there has been a crisis. We have spent our holidays in Raigmore Hospital, Inverness, or visiting his mother in the 'home' whilst his father recovered from an operation. Or shopping, cooking, doing the garden. We have driven his father back and forth from Ullapool to Inverness, sixty miles each way, hospital visiting everyday.

We gave his father every support when he had his operation. We have taken his mother out and sat through difficult visiting times. Wonder what we did wrong? Can't believe father-in-law can be so cruel.

Think that the two sisters, brother-in-law, four grownup grandchildren, including wife and partner can pull their weight now. Don't think that's unreasonable, very cross and upset. Need a second opinion, too near the problem. Ask Beth. Beth said I am to concentrate on getting myself better, nice to have an independent view.

17

THREE MEN IN A BOAT

DISOBEDIENCE

James James, Morrison Morrison Weatherby George Dupree, took great care of his mother, through he was only three. James James said to his mother "Mother," he said, said he; "You must never go down to the end of town if you don't go down with me."

James James Morrison's Mother put on a golden gown, James James Morrison's Mother drove to the end of town.

James James Morrison's mother said to herself, said she: "I can get right down to the end of town and be back in time for tea."

King John put up a notice, "LOST or STOLEN or STRAYED! JAMES JAMES MORRISON'S MOTHER, SEEMS TO HAVE BEEN MISLAID. LAST SEEN WANDERING VAGUELY: QUITE OF HER OWN ACCORD, SHE TRIED TO GET DOWN TO THE END OF THE TOWN--FORTY SHILLINGS REWARD!

James James Morrison Morrison (commonly known as Jim) told his other relations not to go blaming him. James James said to his Mother, "Mother", he said, said he: "You must never go down to the end of town without consulting me."

James James Morrison's mother hasn't been heard of since. King John said he was sorry, so did the Queen and Prince. King John (somebody told me) said to a man he knew: "If people go down to the end of the town, well, what can anyone do?"

J. J. M. M. W. G. Du P, took great C/o of his M***** though he was only 3. J. J. said to his M***** "M*****", he said, said he: "You-must-never-go-down-to-the-end-of-the-town-if-you-don't-go-down-with-ME!"

A. A Milne

I put that in for no other reason than I like it.

18

I seem to have acquired two other survivors in my leaky lifeboat. They are on baling out duties until I can think of a "cunning plan".

A friend of mine, a Norwegian, (a great sailing nation), told me that lifeboats are always picked up. I said I felt as though the big ship was disappearing over the horizon, people waving and saying "be positive". Have to keep morale up, check supplies. Haven't any, check navigation instruments haven't any. Down to our own resources.

One is beginning to waver, try shock tactics, (recycle tactics used on me) and it works. Try some humour at my own expense, seems to work too. Two of us believe in God, one not sure, but likes the idea of being prayed for, says it helps. Find it very strange to be thrown together, all very different types, would never have been friends before, but tolerate each other because we have all been through an awful experience. One says it is exhausting being brave, and has cried once or twice. I say the only time I nearly cried was when people are nice to me. Seems we have all had a rotten time one way or another in our lives and pushed our bodies into second place. We all know what is needed to get our bodies to work properly again and seem to have re-appraised our lifestyle.

Feel if one of us gets better, we all want to get better together. The good wishes and concern for each other, amazes us all, can't believe strangers can be so good to each other. We look at each other and know the other person is in exactly the same position, no false platitudes. One very keen on the internet and technical detail, frightens me a little, don't want to know too much detail, just enough to understand. One very kind about hair loss and always takes her wig off to make me feel better. Her head looks much more beautiful than mine. Compliment her on her twinkley eyes; always think eyes are the most important feature of a person. Can't disguise a person's personality or soul, shows in the eyes.

We have noticed how people respond to us by being much more honest about anything they are talking about. Why should having cancer make people more open about themselves, have been told the most personal and sensitive things by strangers and friends alike. Perhaps they think it doesn't matter because I am on another planet or will not be here long to repeat it. Perhaps it is because they feel guilty or relieved they are not me. I wish I was normal again and blended in with the crowd, not a natural or willing patient.

MY MUM AND MY DAD

THE NAUGHTY BOY

There was a naughty boy,
And a naughty boy was he,
He ran away to Scotland
The people for to see-
Then he found
That the ground
Was as hard,
That a yard
Was as long,
That a song
Was as merry,
That a cherry
Was as red-
That lead
Was as weighty,
That four score
Was as eighty.
That a door
Was as wooden
As in England-
So he stood in his shoes
And he wondered,
He wonder'd,
He stood in his shoes
And he wondered.

John Keats

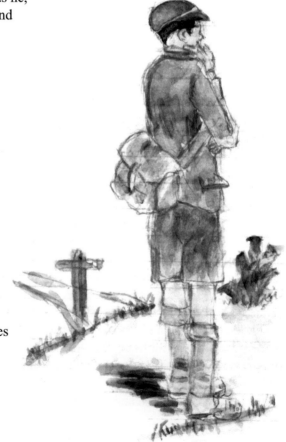

When I was a child I used to sit on the stairs and liked nothing better than to chew on a cheese rind (well there was food rationing then you know) and read this poem, that my mother had found in one of her books. It kept me quiet and I have always thought how true it is, everywhere and everyone basically the same.

When I was small, mothers stayed at home and looked after their children. I wasn't spoilt, but I did have a very happy childhood. Two parents, without two halfpennies to rub together, they gave my sister and I, not things, but their time and attention, their principles.

I ambled through life, not ambitious, not trying hard at anything. Fell into my job by chance, got to like it. Had boyfriends, liked very few really, fended off engagement rings and proposals. Remained on good terms with my parents who were very happy together. Met Malcolm one summer, got engaged at Christmas, everything idyllic, until one day, the consultant told my mother at the garden gate, in passing, that my father would not live until the wedding in July.

My mother devastated, distraught, heartbroken. My father wanting me to look after my mother. Me, about to get married, torn between Malcolm, my sick father and looking after my mother.

My father lived by will power to the wedding; I didn't enjoy my wedding at all, too upset about Dad. Dad lived until October. He knew I would not leave my mother to fend for herself. Made a promise to look after her and 22 years later I am still doing my best to keep that promise.

Get on well with my mother, managed to battle with bureaucrats, insurance officials, tradesmen, fuse-boxes, on her behalf. Always manage to win my battles somehow. Always thought I would be well and strong, as I always have been, everything would be alright because I would always be around to sort it out, keep her independent in her own home. Never liked being ill, never wanted to be ill, didn't realise there was a problem at all, no pain, just felt a little more tired than usual. Insidious cancer, crept upon me, like a cruel joke, don't think you are going to have an easy ride, time you had another nasty shock, let's see how you get out of this one. One battle I can't win on my own.

2003

THIS ENGLISH WOMAN

This English woman is so refined,
She has no bosom and no behind.

Stevie Smith 1902-1971

So what's going to happen? What are the results going to be? Am I going to get a good report, will they be pleased with my progress or will I get a comment like I used to at school 'could do better', 'careless mistakes', 'not working to her potential'. Hopeless at mathematics, trying to work out reduction I think should happen to lumps, after every chemotherapy treatment.

My body started this, so my body can stop it. My body is in a "huff" with me, must be nice to my body.

Sad news at third chemotherapy treatment 30 December 2002, Beth has had an "accident" and has "head injuries", no other details. She had gone on a skiing holiday, jokingly "I said I hoped she wouldn't break a leg"; wished I hadn't said it now. Very shocked and upset and hope she is alright, left message with nurse to give to Jenny, Beth's colleague. Doesn't seem fair that these things happen to the good people and all the bad people seem to get away with it.

Would like to ring and find out how Beth is, but they don't give bad news over the phone and they only tell the truth, so that's not a good idea. Decide not to write another word until I find out how she is.

Plucked up courage and rang Jenny to find out how Beth is doing. Relieved to hear she is going to get better and is improving slowly.

• • • • • •

24/1/2003

After third check-up with Dr. E. which went very well I thought, she said "we're getting there". Jenny, Beth's colleague, came to see me whilst I was tethered to my chemotherapy treatment. Jenny is doing both case

22

loads now so obviously is very busy. She introduced herself and gave me quite a lot of her time. Think I have 'blown it' it with her, complained about being ill and not being able to deal with it myself. Dreadful attitude, double checked liver scan results too, 'Oh dear', started to regress.

· · · · · ·

BONES

Heaven take my soul and England keep my bones!

King John - Shakespeare.

Banged my head on the garage door, saw stars for a few seconds. Nice sunny day thought I'd do a few jobs out in the fresh air, day dreaming and walked into the garage door. Nothing wrong with that bone anyway, just a sore lump, knocked a few more brain cells out, will not be able to understand anything now!

A little worried that Dr. E. would comment on my head bump, but thankfully if she found out from Jenny, she didn't think it important, so I didn't get into trouble for that. I had been very embarrassed last time, trying to wriggle off an uncomfortable hook, explaining my stroppy Sainsbury's episode. Not to mention X-ray department fiasco.

· · · · · ·

HALF-WAY

"No passion so effectually robs the mind of all its powers of acting and reasoning as fear"

On the Sublime and Beautiful. (1757) - Edmund Burke 1729-97

Dr. E. running very late with clinic, but it didn't matter too much as Sue and I were amusing ourselves, looking at my file and book. In fact quite relaxed when she walked in, so much so I forgot myself and said "phew it's hot in here, are you hot or is it me?". Dr. E. surprised me by saying "no she wasn't hot" and explained that she came from a hot country and she had never got used, in 25 years here, of the cold.

Stumped for a reply, I said she was in the wrong country; as it would never be hot here. Then I thought that sounded a little offhand and puzzled which country was so hot. Off on wrong track again.

Dr. E. showed no interest in the lump under my arm and concentrated on the breast lump. She had a very clever trick of comparing pressure reduction by simply looking at bra marks. Something I hadn't thought of and said so, trying to make amends for my comment, "I hadn't thought of that and that she was cleverer that me". Modestly she said "it was 25 years of experience", which made me smile, something I don't normally do when flat on my back being examined. She then said I'd had a tough time, but was getting "there", she was so kind I nearly cried. I was also so pleased with the "getting there" bit, that I instructed Sue to "put that down" in the file, in case I forgot or thought I had imagined it. I added out loud "I'll savour that later". So pleased with that little crumb of comfort.

I had earlier asked for more suppositories please and jokingly added I thought they were wonderful and I had become a suppository bore, they were so much better than the alternative of terrible sickness.

I was also told I would see the surgeon next time (get used to the word) to see "if I am doing a good job". Me "I'm sure you are and most grateful thanks".

Stumped again when asked, "what would I like?" a comment flashed through my head and I stopped myself just in time, Dr. E. must have seen my face change and quickly said "what do you need?" missed the point, couldn't think what to say, what does she mean? Just said I didn't know what I needed. Perhaps she was alluding to Beth not being around any more, I hadn't mentioned it. Said she was moving my appointment to Thursdays, Breast Day. Hurray perhaps I can have a lollipop now, trouble is haven't any mouth ulcers.

JENNY – 1ST RESERVE
1/2003

> ## "Words are, of course, the most powerful drug used by mankind".

Rudyard Kipling

Jenny kindly gave me some of her valuable time on the fourth session; she has two case loads now and must be wandering how she will cope. Hope they don't overwork her. She is young and has magnificent hair and the confidence to wear it, wish I had. Rather vented my frustration at being in my 'hole' of my own making. Also made clear "we don't like theorists, do we Sue?" So I didn't expect she will be back, why should she, I made it clear I wasn't bothered either way. Very naughty and ungrateful. Still there are plenty of people who will appreciate her help and need it more than me. Tried to make amends by recalling some antics of the children at school and said I had worked with behaviour problems so long I had become one myself. Hope she has a sense of humour or we are in for a very dull time! She is only young and no doubt knows her job better than I do. Take 100 lines "I must not be stroppy" and add 100 lines "I must not whinge". Stop being ungrateful, the only person responsible for the hole I am in is me. I am cross with myself for being so stupid as to have put myself in a hole and now have to accept good people's time, expertise and NHS money to get me out of it.

· · · · · ·

SEVERAL
13/2/2003

Definition of several: - Three or more.

> ## If we see light at the end of the tunnel, it's the light of the oncoming train.

Robert Lowell

TIMETABLE

The Cavalry came, then the Lancers, then the Royal Engineers.

(Malcolm's magnetron)

THE SURGEON
5/2/2003

"When you are a Bear of Very Little Brain, and you Think of things, you find sometimes that a Thing which seemed very Thingish inside you is quite different when it gets out into the open and has other people looking at it."

A.A Milne 1882-1956 The House at Pooh Corner (1928).

• • • • • •

I like that designation, "Surgeon", short and to the point.

No misunderstanding there. As usual, getting into nervous mode for a consultation. Do some painting in my 'booket' to calm me down, brush in mid air when wafting over from the radio is a request from a Beth from Lincolnshire, a song from Sibelious's Finlandia 'Be still my heart' beautifully sung by a Welsh choir, as if by magic, I'm calm. Sail through surgeon's appointment "very good progress", no radiotherapy, just an operation. Float home, still calm even though operation was mentioned. Think might be able to tackle next Dr. E. consultation without so many nerves. Mammogram, Ultrasound at end of sixth chemotherapy "still calm".

MY NURSE, SARAH

> **"In the face of such overwhelming statistical possibilities, hypochondria has always seemed to me to be the only rational position to take on life"**

(1998) John Diamond. Because Cowards Get Cancer Too.

All in white, I wonder where she keeps her wings. I expect modern wings are like some anoraks that fold up really small and as if by magic disappear into a small pocket, ready for instant action if need be. Sarah has a sense of humour thank goodness and doesn't mind listening to my awful stories about school and the children. Very busy and doing a very responsible job well. At my first session she obviously wanted it to go well first time, but even though I didn't look, (it's off putting when someone is watching) also I didn't want to go wobbly. The needle didn't go into the vein quite right, I had been told I had good veins. (good for something then) she apologised and had to ask the "boss", felt sorry for her, although that didn't stop me checking, the drugs etc. reminding her I was having bone drug etc, etc. Just what she needed, a control freak. Got in a complete muddle with the pill instruction, had to get Veronica to write it down.

Sarah tried hard to do her, "some people keep a diary", "it helps with the side-effects". "*SIDE EFFECTS*" not me I'm not having those, "its helps to visualise my washing away the bad cells" *WASH AWAY *", I don't do Airy Fairy wash away. She will be telling me to be "POSITIVE" next, yes like winning the Lottery. Bad enough not being allowed to drive, Beth said it slows you down. I've news for Beth it doesn't it speeds you up. (I'll write about the white van and the big red van when the Police have lost interest.)

Keep forgetting I'm tethered and wave my arm about making the bleeper sound. Feel really spoilt, cups of tea, biscuits, sandwiches at lunch time, and I've heard about the 'ice-lollies' determined to have a mouth ulcer to qualify.

Decide Sarah needs a medal for putting up with me.

TIPS FOR WIG WEARERS

(Rhyming Slang- Syrup of Fig, Wig)

1) Don't garden near rose bushes wearing your wig.

2) If bothered by Double Glazing salesmen etc. just answer the door, smile and take your wig off.

3) Be positive about a visit from the Jehovah's witnesses, they will pray for you.

4) When deliverymen, deposit new furniture in your house and try to escape without assembling it, just say, yes I do want it put together, I'm not doing it, I've got cancer. No problem, quick assembly, in silence.

5) When waiting in a queue at the chemists, behind someone wanting a remedy for a "dying man who has a cold", suggest chemotherapy readjustment wig, and go to front of queue.

6) Make sure that the neighbour whom you can't get on with, sees you being very active e.g. cleaning windows, walking to post-box etc. with your woolly hat on.

7) Don't adjust your wig in the car mirror when driving.

• • • • • •

14/3/2003

Sandra leading lady, lead us thro' thus lachrymose labyrinth. Or "Just a moment whilst I wash the soap".

Well that's alright, it is only a dream, I'm Alice in Wonderland. Corridors, people in white coats, rooms getting smaller, me getting bigger, tables going up and down. It's very hot, it's not hot, confusion, tablets medicine, equipment, blacked out windows, words meaning what you choose them to mean.

Talk of tattoos, -it's no good being affronted about having or not having a tattoo; if you wanted an ice lolly. Not logical.

Who is telling you to "be calm" just before your visit to the surgeon? Anodyne words or a kick up the pants? Which will work, -both for me.

Salvage some pride and independence for goodness sake, get your own booklets.

14/3/2003
BELL, BOOK AND CANDLE

Ironic isn't it? I used to work on the site of the medical Leper Colony in Lincoln. Now I'm the one with a disease. Dr. Several has taken my candle, I've got a book (booket really) and I used to go bell ringing. Shall I be a bell ringing bore and explain how bell ringing is done, not just the mechanics, but have you ever wondered how the ringers ring their bells without memorising a list of place numbers? I can see your eyes glazing over, but it is very interesting and not a little clever. Especially for someone hopeless at maths like me. Ironic too, that if I have radiotherapy it will probably be from a valve (power source) that Malcolm was responsible for R' & D'ing. He is not too happy about this, too much responsibility. Malcolm, by the way has a PhD in Hypochondria and is nearly cured, wish I was. Not really, its in low temperature magnetism.

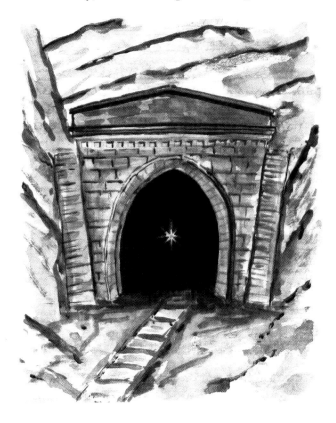

PART 2

WHEN, NOT IF.
RENAMED 'MY BOOK OF BURBLING'S.

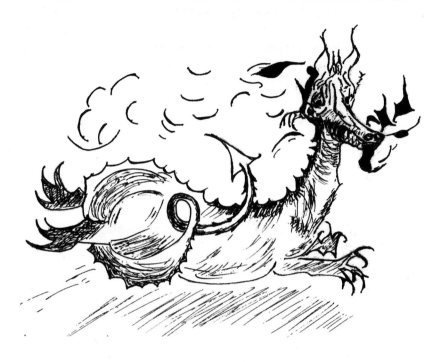

THE CAGE

It tried to get out of the cage;
Here and there it ran, and tried
At the edges and the side,
In a busy, timid rage.

Trying yet to find the key
Into freedom, trying yet,
In a timid rage, to get
To its old tranquillity.

It did not know, it did not see,
It did not turn an eye, or care
That a man was watching there
While it raged so timidly.

It ran without a sound, it tried,
In a busy, timid rage,
To escape from out the cage
By the edges and the side.

James Stephens 1882 -1950

• • • • • •

CURIOSITY KILLED THE CAT.
15/3/2003

"Beware the Ides of March", Malcolm's birthday 15th March. A fatal day from the prophetic warning, said to have been given to Julius Caesar.

Why do I have this insatiable curiosity? It always gets me into trouble.

What is that grey box of electrical equipment in the consulting room and what's in the long box that looks like a musical instrument? What are those numbers behind the desk, on the wall in the waiting room?

I'd much rather talk about the <u>C</u> word climate, than the <u>C</u> word cancer.

Talking of C words, I'd like to tell you about the Condensed Milk. We had to do the washing-up when I was at Primary School, I would be about seven or eight years old and the teachers had a hot drink at playtime. We, who stayed for lunch, sandwiches, because we lived too far away to walk home and back in time for afternoon school, didn't get a hot drink all day. This didn't seem to bother the teachers in the winter and the winters were twice as cold as they are now.

However, the point is, if you leave a tin of condensed milk open near a child who takes her ration book to the sweet shop, you can hardly be surprised if she sticks her finger into it, goodness knows where my finger had been.

I told my father, because I never learnt guile and he made me eat a whole tin, I have never eaten any since.

Why is it that whenever I mention that "I have written about you in my booket", people become very defensive for absolutely no reason at all?

Now, I know, as a teacher, I spent my life writing notes and reports, making quick judgements, sometimes incorrectly, mostly very near the mark.

So, if you leave my notes rolled up at my chemotherapy treatment machine I will look at them, it will not do me any good at all, but I will not resist the temptation! Similarly, if I get into curiosity, questioning mode, I will not stop until I have heard what I do not want to know. I wish it had been Beth there and not Dr. Several. She would not have allowed me to wind myself up, she would have called me Susan, not Sue and I would have known I had over stepped the mark.

It has taken nearly four months, three people, to wear down my resistance to my conscience. I wish I didn't have one; it would be so much easier. Tackled the easy problems first, easy to see, not so easy to tackle but we did it, Malcolm and I. Now I'm down to the really hard problems. Malcolm and God are working on these. I have no idea how I am going to solve them. Was it stupid to try and solve them? Was it stupid to try and do my best, do the right thing? Would I do the same again? Thank you Sue and Sarah.

A TESTING TIME
K. B. O
19/3/2003
PART 1

> ## "I'm afraid you've got a bad egg Mr. Jones. Oh no, my Lord, I assure you! Parts of it are excellent!"

Punch 1895.

A nice touch that, warming the gel for the Ultrasound scan. Getting quite blasé about undressing now, not too bothered how many people look at me. Alison the nurse quite concerned I was well covered up for the dash across the corridor to the other consulting room, where Malcolm was waiting. Kept blessing me, she must have been nervous, well I'll take as many blessings as are offered to me thank you.

Apologised to Jenny for whinging, she said she couldn't remember me doing it, but I knew otherwise. Said I had heard Beth's request on Classic FM. Jenny said she didn't know about it, but said Beth liked classical music. I said, "I had better be careful as we weren't allowed to talk about Beth and I would get a lecture on patient confidentiality". At least she saw the funny side of that comment.

Professor E. came in just as I was sharing some hand cream with Malcolm, so he had difficulty shaking his hand and I was sorry I had embarrassed Malcolm by being naughty again.

Professor E. launched into a complicated explanation of the pros and cons of the next lot of treatment. Radiotherapy had obviously been already decided, despite Dr. Several's comments earlier, talk about confusing the patient. So there I am calmly or trying to, calmly talk about whether I am to be shot or hung.

Dr. E. came in and made a comment about Malcolm having the Red File today. I feel hemmed in with three on one side and Malcolm and I listening with our backs to the wall.

Liked the way Dr. E. stood her ground when questioned by Prof. E. his manner is friendly and confident, but I think I prefer Dr. E's way, less words, difficult to say, if anyone is really on our side, however much Prof. E. tries to be friendly. I think he is quite capable of making a hard decision with a smile. The strain of the day, two appointments and waiting, plus the awful seriousness of the consultation begins to take its toll on my patience. Prof. E. wants to examine me, Jenny comes forward and seems to confront me and I explode with my frustration at being misled about Bone Disease expectation. Feel let down, and angry. Jenny makes excuses for me about being stressed etc, etc. I say no, they are my blasted bones and it wasn't fair and "I had done it again".

Prof. E. emerges, all soothing words now he thinks the explosion is over, "good sign the first one had gone quickly".

Dr. E. had earlier said I had had a "good response" to the chemotherapy. Goodness knows what is going to be decided. I feel cornered, no control over my life or what is to happen to it. Jenny comments on the Red File "says it's a good idea as I put the prescription away". I say "it's my attempt to control the uncontrollable".

· · · · · ·

EPIGRAMS
20/3/2004

RELATIVITY

There was a young woman named Bright
Who travelled much faster than light,
She started one day
In the relative way, and returned on the preceding night.

Anonymous

· · · · · ·

34

MIND OVER MATTER

There was a faith healer of Deal
Who said "Although pain isn't real,
If I sit on a pin
And it punctures my skin
I dislike what I fancy I feel" .

Anonymous

FREE WILL AND PREDESTINATION

There was a young man who said "Damn!
It appears to me now that I am
Just a being that moves
In predestinate grooves-
Not a bus, not a bus, but a tram."

Maurice Hare

• • • • • •

My candle burns at both ends;
It will not last the night;
But ah, my foes, and oh, my friends-
It gives a lovely light!

Edna St. Vincent Millay

RADIOTHERAPY
27/30/2003

(RAP)

Radiotherapy, classic or three,
Relax to the music of therapy.

Pristine machine,
Room light and clean,
Relax to the music of therapy.

Lined and "lay still",
Say Sue, Jan and Jill,
Relax to the music of therapy.

Out shoot the rays,
Extending my days,
Relax to the music of therapy.

Slap on the cream,
The swelling can't be seem,
Relax to the music of therapy.

We thought she was potty,
But she's only dotty*,
Relax to the music of therapy.

* read 'Tattoos'
S. Scouller

"LET'S MAKE NO BONES ABOUT IT"
2/4/2003

"When I use a word", Humpty Dumpty said in rather a scornful tone, "it means just what I choose it to mean-neither more nor less".

"The question is", said Alice, "whether you can make words mean so many different things".

"The question is", said Humpty Dumpty, "which is to be Master-that's all".
Alice was too much puzzled to say anything, so after a minute Humpty Dumpty began again. "They've a temper, some of them-particularly verbs, they're the proudest-adjectives you can do anything with, but not verbs-however, I can manage the whole lot of them! Impenetrability! That's what I say".

Through the Looking Glass, Lewis Carroll.

· · · · · ·

CALLED
"POOLE AND DON'T FORGET THE BLASTED E."

She promised to be good,
In everyway she could,
But she forgot her name.

She wondered if she should,
Revert to Sue, she would
But like to hear her name.
Sue.

37

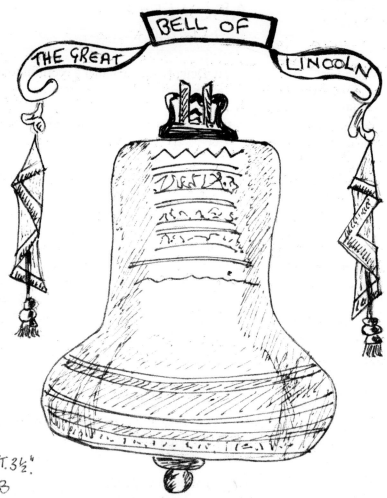

THE GREAT BELL OF LINCOLN

DIA. 6 FT. 3½"
NOTE B

3 TONS
18 CWT.
3 QR 18 lbs.

'GREAT TOM' 1610

A TESTING TIME
PART 2

2/4/2003

Another hot day, Malcolm said I had a red mark on my neck, coming out in blotches, Dr. E. walked in took one look at me and opened the window. Bone scan results are not there so everyone goes out again.

We all start again, a nurse comes in and I said "reinforcements", Prof. E. smiled at that, I think they are expecting trouble. Prof. E. said bones haven't spread, but that's all they could say, which is what Dr. E. said last time; will have to wait six months. Operation is off and its radiotherapy, they seem surprised I think the tattoos a good idea. Everyone out again, nurse positions herself in front of me and looks into my eyes, whilst chewing gum, which rather distracts me, I hope she doesn't swallow it. I said I feel "trapped like a wild animal you take to the vet and have to inject to get near it to treat it". Nurse goes out Dr. E. back in or was she there all the time, so much to-ing and froing. I say my bit about "not wanting to be shunted into a siding because of my bones". "If I hung about something might turn up and I was going to hang about anyway to be awkward". Dr. E. said I wasn't being shunted and seemed optimistic, I got a hug around the shoulders which surprised me, trying to cheer me up I suppose. Said we might as well get on with the radiotherapy, (no point in arguing). I think they were expecting me to explode again and seemed relieved the "wild animal" was docile. Another hug to cheer me up. I think they got away very lightly.

Go home to read my new book, "Love, Medicine and Miracles" by Bernie Siegel MD my little ray of light. Have a major wobble, keep reading the book. Booked reflexology session, but get muddled and call it refluxology which means I think being sick.

REFLEXOLOGY
OR CHINESE FOOTSIE
17/4/2003

Tread carefully,
Tip-toe round my toes.
Round and round it goes.

Creaming, smoothing pressure,
One at once and two together
Stroking with a feather.

Let's stay like this for ever,
Mind floating in a trance….
…like a foot flexing dance.

I have been looking forward to my reflexology session, having had a good recommendation from Irene. She said she loves it and she sees colours in her minds eye. So I'm very keen to see colours too. Soothing, relaxing music is playing, fill in the questionnaire, no; I don't have any trouble with my bowels. I have come to be calmed down at the other end of my body, the part most dear to me, my mind. Lie down on the bed, feet wiped with a tissue and the session begins. Like it, straight away. Very gentle pressure sends my brain into a trance that I don't want to go to leave. I don't want to go to sleep I might miss some of that lovely trance like "Alpha" state feeling. I've got the jargon now. Alpha state is the first level of hypnosis, so I've read in my new book.

Looking forward to my next session, I'm having six sessions and all on the NHS, an excellent idea. I think I am becoming addicted to relaxation. Dictate a visualisation tape for myself for meditation. Have to redo it because I sneeze halfway through! Try it out and fall asleep somewhere near the end so it must have worked.

RADIOTHERAPY

5/5/2003

> **Now here you see, it takes all the running you can do, to keep in the same place. If you want to get somewhere else, you must run at least twice as fast as that!**

Lewis Carroll - 'Through the Looking Glass'

Issued with my 'activity sheet', I arrive for my daily dose (for five weeks) and wait, and wait and wait. Really tired and bored, missed my 9.30am session, still haven't seen Dr. E. apparently, big mix-up, they think I haven't signed the consent form, I with a flourish produce from the "RED FILE" the said form, can't resist saying it "pays to be organised". My Red File was useful after all. Manage to keep my patience with everyone and have first session. Three very nice people set up the machine match up lines to the information on the two TV screens. Very difficult to relax, close my eyes and wait for the machine to work. Feel a sinking sensation, maybe my imagination. Told to get up, but they forgot to untie my arm.

On my third Activity Sheet now, due to mistakes about Bank Holidays.

Put onto different machine LA3; discover the Magnetron was one designed by Malcolm, now made in Chelmsford.

The department has walls five foot and three foot thick because of the radiation. I keep my own gown for changing into everyday.

Alison and the A Team, Andrew and another Alison are very good, Alison explains all the numbers on the screen to me and I watch as the numbers all correspond correctly as they move the bed up and down, back and forwards to a very small tolerance.

To make life more interesting, we start to think of themes. I said I felt like Cleopatra and they could bring me wine and grapes, Alison a good sport, warms to the theme and said Asses milk too. So I designate each one a role, Mark Anthony etc. StarTreck is the next one with the Time Machine, Captain Kirk etc. The student is looking a little bemused at all of this, not sure if we should be joking or not.

Seem to be getting used to the therapy, quite tired the first few weeks, but now, quite normal, been for long walks when ever possible. Sister on Ingham Ward said I must have the constitution of an Ox, which I will take as a compliment. Skin a little red, but nothing painful, hoping for a good report on Friday for Exit Review. Feel quite calm, so maybe the reflexology is working. Have my radiotherapy review and Zometa all on Friday morning. Have a chat with Sarah who always seems to unhook me from the 'drip', report bone scan news, she is pleased.

There is an unspoken camaraderie, amongst everyone going for treatment, people look at you and you know what they are thinking. Everyone gives each other a smile and encouraging word. Old hands trying to help and cheer up the new worried ones.

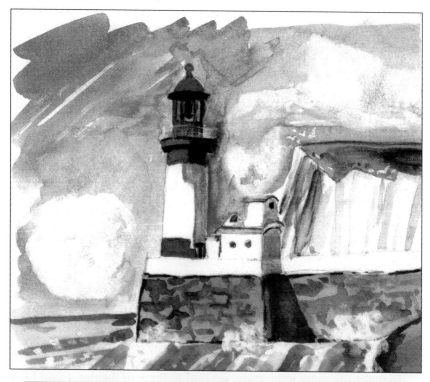

"It is not in the still calm of life, or the repose of a pacific station, that great characters are formed... Great necessities call out great virtues."

Abigail Adams 1744-1818

THE BAG LADY
(WITH THE RED FILE)
25/5/2003

Reverting back to what I know in a crisis, I have always taken my Red File and various things pen, diary, car-park money, banana in case of famine, a general life support system, with me, all in a very sturdy, capacious 'Lakeland' plastic bag.

When ever I go to the hospital, this goes with me. I think it's a good idea nothing gets lost, its all there somewhere. The Red File has all my letters, reference numbers, notes, consent forms (proved useful as described earlier).

I know I am only doing what the children at school did, taking my security blanket. One of my friends said I could have as many 'props' as I liked, so I will and blow what people think. Anyway they recognise me now by my bag. I'm the lady with the Lakeland bag. I put in a book of poetry I got for my birthday. It is so much better trying to get to grips with Milton than staring at the wall.

I'm trying an experiment next appointment with Dr. E. I'm going to see if I dare go without my wig. My hair is growing back and I quite like the feel of it on top of my head. When I stroke it, it feels like a mole's pelt or a cat's fur. I've got used to seeing myself and my real hair colour dark brown, and I've got my eyebrows and lashes back too.

No self-respecting cancer would want to be seen dead with anyone looking like I do at the moment. So I'm hoping it will go away, that's the theory.

I think I might be in trouble again. Last Zometa I went for a walk between radiotherapy and Zometa appointment. I like to get exercise and fresh air, walked all round the hospital perimeter. At my Exit appointment with Dr. E. I was surprised when she came into the waiting room, looking for me. Now I know why Sandra came up to me, when I was hooked up and asked if I wanted to see Dr. E., last time I was alright. I thought I just went thro' to Ingham ward and got my dose. I think they think I've skipped classes. I got my hand smacked too for touching my skin when Dr. E. checked it at the end of radiotherapy. She told me not to rub it or touch it and course I did. She gave me some cream and dressings. The worst part of the sore skin was after a shower, I found a cool block from the freezer was the only thing which stopped the itching. Try getting a cool block wedged into your bra, it's not easy.

Took a thank you card and a small bunch of flowers to Anne on last reflexology session. I scoured my garden for a rose and the only one out didn't have any scent. So I found a beautiful scented one sticking out of some railings on a building site. Anne very pleased and I've got an "ology" now!

• • • • • •

NON-STANDARD
26/5/2003

Is it very mystical?
To be so un-statistical?

It's not a very nice name,
I'd rather be the same.

I'm sure they would not mind,
Are there many of my kind?

I think it's very lonely,
To be a one and only.

Please let me join the others too,
A group of Standard and a Sue!

S. Scouller

Dr. E. does not want to see me six weeks after the Radiotherapy as stated in the leaflet. She said I am "Non Standard".

• • • • • •

FRIENDS

Walk with me,
Talk with me,
Be there with me.

S. Scouller

My friends are still with me, they have not faded seven months after this nightmare started. They are loyal, good, kind, decent people, every one of them.

• • • • • •

BAG LADY

They call her the 'bag lady'.
Put it down for a while.
That bag and that Red File.
"I'll put it down, maybe."

What do you need it for?
It has no use anymore,
That bag and that Red File.
"I'll put it down, when I am well, maybe."

You know it is just a prop.
I bet it weighs a lot,
That bag and that Red File.
"I will put it down, one day soon, ………… maybe."

S. Scouller

The nurses in Ingham Ward identified me as the Lady with the Lakeland Bag, when I went for my six Chemo' sessions. I always have it with me when I go to hospital. I have been teased about it and my Red File too. Now my hair is starting to grow back slowly they will not recognise me without it. I can go incognito, not such a silly idea!

45

A HAIRY QUESTION
OR A SHORT CUT TO AN ANSWER!
26/5/2003

Has anyone seen my hair?
I left it hanging....where?
I wonder if I dare,
Will people look and stare?
If I go out without my hair.

I've been looking for my hair,
It was on the bedpost there.
Will my head be cold and bare?
Oh! I really do not care,
If I go out without my hair.

S. Scouller

My hair is about half an inch long all over now, I'm not sure if it is greyer than before. People don't seem to notice it when I go out; I think there are so many styles these days. They probably think I am just an ageing punk. I wonder if I am brave enough to go on Friday without my hair?

· · · · · ·

A PAIN IN THE NECK
5/6/2003

"life is just one damned thing after another."

Elbert Hubbard.

November 4th 2002 I was due to go to Nottingham City Hospital for a right Thyroidectomy (hemi) after waiting about nine months for the operation. About two weeks before I went for my routine three year Breast screening check and treatment for Breast Cancer was

46

started straight away. The thyroid has been in the pending file ever since. No point seeing the thyroid consultant whilst having Chemo' or Radiotherapy. Now that there is a lull in proceedings I fitted in a check up at Nottingham City Hospital.

Mr. U. said I should have an operation in the next month and he would write to Lincoln and consult with them. So I have to get my operation done between Zometa appointments and I was so looking forward to swimming and bell ringing again. Mr. U. said it was very rare, this circumstance, Malcolm said he seemed quite excited about the operation and I repeated the 'non standard' explanation, which he raised his eyebrows to and so did I.

Have kitted myself out with a walkman radio/tape player. I can now listen to music in the waiting room plus take my Visualisation and Meditation and favourite music tapes to hospital.

I hope I can go for walks around the hospital grounds; I want to keep up my exercise. I am trying not to think about the results of any tests they will do. It is a bit much trying to fight on two fronts at once. Maybe someone will say what the plan is going to be now. If anyone asks me how I am I say "alright so far thank you".

· · · · · ·

KOO CUT
5/7/2003

"Oh Lord! Thou knowest how busy I must be this day if I forget thee, do not thou forget me". Jacob Astley 1579-1652. Before the Battle of Edgehill......... and my........... OPERATION JULY 8th TUESDAY 2003 approx 12.00-2.00pm.

Koo Stark is in the paper, I see she has copied my hair style with a crew-cut. It suits her and she looks very well after treatment. Hope my hair looks alright, Veronica has given me strict instructions not to touch it and is going to sort it out for me and is insisting on ears being pierced too. Some one said at least my ears, don't stick out! My dentist said, I looked ok, pity about the DODGY hair-cut!

Have had my pre-op checks at Nottingham City Hospital. Mr. U. is going to do the operation himself, so that's good. Have to ring Monday morning to check I have a bed and operation on Tuesday. Want to get on

47

with it now and get the results.

Went down to Branston Church to see my bell ringing friends and they all came to see me. Christopher had saved all the Ringing World papers and guild booklets for me, paid my £6 Guild subscription in April (that's faith for you!) plus latest quarter peal certificate for me for my last quarter peal at Metheringham before I became ill last November. Added a photograph and the most touching thing of all that they could have done, on Thursday practise night I missed because I was at the hospital being given BAD NEWS, they rang a quarter peal and dedicated to me for "a speedy recovery". How is that for kindness?

Christopher (he is 17 years old now and I have known him since he was 11 years) showed me photographs of the new bells they have got for Potterhanworth Church, only £5000 to raise now for a new frame. He said I am to be in the team that first rings six bells at Potterhanworth for about two hundred years. They have only three now, not enough for method ringing.

STEAK AND THYROID PIE

8/7/2003

> ## "You should make a point of trying every experience once, excepting incest and folk-dancing".

Anonymous

I can recommend Nottingham City Hospital for a relaxing holiday, good food, excellent room service, good varied company.

I am soon institutionalised, with my Thrombosis socks, on and hospital gown, like a large pretty J Cloth. Observations done and an injection in my stomach. Blood oxygen level 99% very good. Thermometer stuck in my ear and blood pressure taken.

My neighbours are a heroin*, alcoholic, cannabis, twenty a day smoker on morphine whose bed looks like a disaster area, and an eighty six year old lady emergency ulcer admission. *Thank-goodness!!*

Find I am quite tired, enjoy the hot milky Ovaltine, have a shower and go to sleep. Lights out about 11.30pm. The ward goes quiet and soon everyone is asleep. About three night staff are on patrol. Cup of tea at 6.00am and then nothing, and wait for trolley. Student Nurse Michael has a chat and is going to be with me all the time and watch the operation. Also Mr. U. asks if a medical student may watch too. Had an idea for raising money for NHS, Videos at say £100 of your operation and £10 for music of your choice to be played!

Pushed down on trolley and parked in front of a small TV on the wall. Start to get bored. More paperwork, labels etc. Mr. U. in his kit comes to say hello with a nice smile. An anaesthetist pushes me through to Bijou theatre 7, my curiosity, distracts me, another girl anaesthetist is waiting, they get to work, hooking me up, plonk me on the table. Doing really well, not wobbling at all, manage a joke. Right leg starts to shake, can't stop it, hope no one sees it, don't want to be a wimp. Anaesthetist says she is giving me something which will relax me, similar to having a Gin and Tonic, good sense of humour and very competent. Go nice and whoozy - fall asleep. No dreams, nothing. Thank goodness, got there at last, at least Nottingham thinks I am worth an operation, very happy thought.

BOOK 3

14/7/2003

This is my new book, reader, a birthday present. It is much smarter than the two tatty exercise books I used before. I feel I must write really smartly, no mistakes, and be very tidy. I am using the pen that goes with it, made out of natural stick.

· · · · · ·

OPERATION CONTINUED.

Brown eyes is calling my name and Michael is looking at me, please go away I don't want to wake up. What is all that noise, I thought wards were supposed to be quiet. Stop asking questions, I'm going to be sick, I am sick, Oh! the pain, give it a score from 1-10? Its 7, my neck, give me a pillow for my neck, to prop it up, please. Brown eyes consults with a nurse, I'm going to have some morphine and anti-sickness drug. The morphine works straight away. I stop climbing out of the bed, over the rails. The nurse brings a hot blanket to put over me and I calm down and go to sleep when she says she will not leave me.

I wake up in the ward, Michael still with me doing the observations; they were done every ten minutes in the recovery ward, now every twenty minutes. I have a drip and spare cannula in my hand, a drain tube and bottle tied to the bed rail, and an oxygen mask on.

Malcolm arrives and looks anxious; I think I am not a pretty sight! Has he put the milk money out? I try to speak but my voice has gone croaky. I am allowed a small cup of water and a straw. Very tired but want to talk to Malcolm he goes away for a sandwich and comes back later at 6pm. Nurses give me painkillers and I try to get out of bed forgetting I'm tied to the rails. My neighbour spots this and helps me to walk wobbly to the lavatory, legs feel like jelly. Have a good nights sleep, still doped. They have moved my bed from no.6 to no.3. They have moved my bedside table and very thin anorexic locker. It is so thin I can only put my shoes away in tandem.

NOTTINGHAM CITY HOSPITAL
8/7/2003

All alone and a long way from home.
I try to speak but it comes out a squeak,
A gun* at my head and rails to my bed,
Tubes and a mask,
The nurse has a task,
Mr U. thought I could cope,
He gave me lots of hope.

* thermometer
S. Scouller.

I'm so pleased to have my Brownie Ops Badge. I'm going to put it under my Chemo' and Radiotherapy Badges. I have a necklace of staples in my neck about twelve, they use glue as well. I can walk about in my dressing gown if I put the drain bottle in my pocket. Walk past a baby, who takes one look at me and starts to cry!

• • • • • •

GOOD NEWS
18/7/2003

Rang Mr. U. secretary and she told me "no evidence of malignancy".

• • • • • •

THE LOOK BOOK
15/8/2003

I'm thinking of writing a book about looks. I have become an expert at looks given to me and their interpretation.

51

Starting with the:-

a) "what's the matter with her, she looks awful" look.
b) "are you here too", look.
c) "are you going to lose your temper", look
d) "I think she's gone potty", look.
e) "what a pity", look.
f) "you can do it", look.
g) "I didn't recognise you without your hair", look.
h) "what on earth is she talking about", look.
i) "humour her", look.
j) "I can't see the join", look.
k) "you still here", look.
l) "she looks too old to have a punk haircut", look.
m) "I expected her to look much worse", look.
n) " hello, it's nice to see you", look (my favourite).

· · · · · ·

MY TEAM

Saw Dr. Several at my pre-op Zometa appointment. I asked lots of questions and called him to task, about misleading me about an operation and another upsetting comment. In fact I gave him quite a grilling. He didn't really have an answer, think I put him on the defensive, anyway got it off my chest (sorry about that). I felt a bit sorry for him in the end and said I only had good people in my team, so if he wanted to be in my team he had to be good and shook hands with him and said goodbye on a friendly note.

Beginning to think I have "powers". I discover at next months Zometa that Dr. Several has left. "Give him a pep talk and he has gone", I said to Sarah in mock amazement.

I had had a little wobble when the thyroid operation was organised, although I wanted to get it done and out of the way, I didn't want to face the test results. I had doubts about my ability to cope with more bad news and more treatment if any. I tried not to allow myself any thoughts about what I should do or not do. I made a 'thank-you' card for Sarah, who had been so very good at talking me out of the "doldrums" and left it with her friend Chris. Sarah's words had been as important to my "response" as any medicine. I couldn't bring myself to actually write thank-you which is what I meant, so I coded it, with a lighthouse picture, a quote from Kilping and called it an un-birthday card to make it light hearted. I thought Sarah was intelligent enough to understand my mind.

I have decided not to say anything at the hospital, about Malcolm losing his job on Friday 13th June, it sounds so improbable they probably would not believe me. I did tell Jenny in my phone call, when I asked for help with a reply to Mr. U. questions which Lincoln took so long to deal with, more excuses. Jenny always looks at me with question marks in her eyes, she probably didn't believe me either, thought I was being dramatic and not up to an operation; not the right one, but an operation and for once, the result was a good one.

· · · · · ·

POST-OP. CHECK-UP NOTTINGHAM
21/8/2003

Mr. U. clinic running about one and half hours late. Saw a nice young man, who seemed pleased with the way my neck had healed. Checked my voice was improving and asked about my bowels. Why is every one so interested in my bowel movements? Felt like saying "fine, how are yours?"! Have to have a small dose of thyroxin, to top up my own supply as I am on the borderline to have it. Checked pre-op blood test results, calcium in my blood within normal range 2.48 (2.2 - 2.6), liver and kidneys alright, good results, I thought, will check Lincoln blood test results at next months Zometa session. It will be interesting to see the calcium level in my blood, post op. Hair out of control now, definitely curly. Dr. E. said it would be.

· · · · · ·

A BIOLOGY LESSON
28/8/2003

T-lymphocytes attack and destroy cancer cells.

Lymphocytes- B & T lymphocytes, formed in the lymphatic system, recognises and helps to destroy invaders and cancer cells. These are both white blood cells.

Interferon produced in response to a cancer cell activates T-lymphocyte.

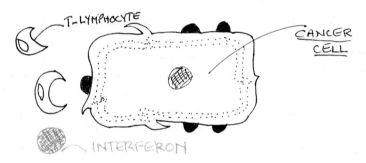

T-lymphocyte attacks and destroys the cancer cell.

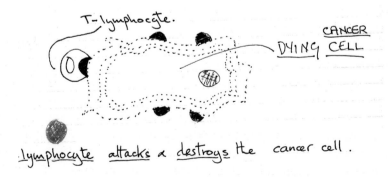

Interferon is a natural protein that limits viral infection by inhibiting viral replication within body cells. These substances also assist in the destruction of cancer cells. The Immune system relies on different types of white blood cells, produced in the lymph glands and bone marrow.

Blood is made up of fifty percent blood cells - red and white and platelets; the remainder is plasma, a straw coloured fluid. Forty percent of the cells are red, white cells and platelets make up about five percent of the total volume. White blood cells are bigger than red blood cells, but much less numerous.

WATCH OUT TIGER T-CELLS ARE ABOUT!

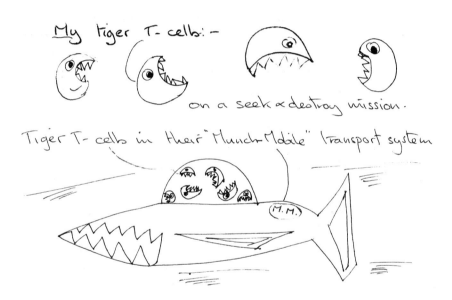

I am concentrating on producing enough Tiger T-cells to destroy all my cancer cells. They whiz up and down my blood stream in their Munch-mobile seeking out the enemy. Munch-mobile is a mini-submarine capable of transporting billons of T-cells. I have billons of mini-submarines too. They look very frightening to the enemy, but they are efficient at their job and are on my side, working for me. They work day and night. Their whole mission in life is to defend me from the enemy--CANCER (cowardly custard). They have all got medals for bravery!

55

BE STILL MY SOUL
6/9/2003

Be still, my soul: the Lord is at your side;
Bear patiently the cross of grief and pain;
Leave to your God to order and provide;
In every change he faithful will remain.
Be still, my soul: your best, your heavenly friend,
Through thorny ways, leads to a joyful end.

Be still, my soul: your God will undertake;
To guide the future as he has the past.
Your hope, your confidence let nothing shake,
All now mysterious shall be clear at last.
Be still, my soul: the tempests still obey
His voice, who ruled them once on Galilee.

Be still, my soul: the hour is hastening on
When we shall be for ever with the Lord,
When disappointment, grief and fear are gone,
Sorrow forgotten, love's pure joy restored.
Be still, my soul: when change and tears are past,
All safe and blessed we shall meet at last.

Hymn from Finlandia. By Sielious. - Beth's request on Classic FM.

Barbara, the wife of my bell ringing team captain found these words for me, it is one of her favourites too. Raymond asked me to help out and ring for a wedding on Saturday 2.30pm. I must get my brains working and look up the methods.

BREAD MAKING, BEEKEEPING AND BELL-RINGING

When I retired I said I wanted to start bread making, so they gave me a bread maker as a leaving present and it has been very good fun too.

I like the idea of beekeeping, but to be practical I don't think the neighbours would appreciate it very much and having been chased up the garden by a swarm of very angry wasps and been stung in sundry places I decided to forego that idea.

So it came to bell ringing. You may have wondered why I put in a picture of 'Great Tom' in booket Part 2. I can hear this wonderful bell chiming the hours when I am at the hospital. I leant to ring when I was about eleven years old and have been pleased to come back to it for the millennium and carried on because of the enthusiasion of Christopher who has over taken me in his skill and expertise. I have only rung once since November 2002 before my op. and Raymond had the good idea of easing me back with a wedding. I like doing these, everyone happy and a traditional event in the village. They are different these days, the "Two for the price of One", amused me. They christened the toddler after the wedding, but at least the little boy was christened. Bells are baptised, named and blessed too.

$$\bullet\ \bullet\ \bullet\ \bullet\ \bullet\ \bullet$$

LOVE IS BLIND,-FRIENDS TURN A BLIND EYE.
8/9/2003

"Oh, the comfort - the inexpressible comfort of feeling safe with a person, having neither to weigh thoughts, nor measure words, but pouring them all out, just as they are, chaff and grain together, knowing that a faithful hand will take and sift them - keep what is worth keeping - and with the breath of kindness blow the rest away."

Anonymous.

MY FOUL WEATHER FRIENDS

Friends - don't ask what they can do, they just do it.
Friends - stay with you in the 'lions' den' (consulting room).
Friends - don't mind if you lose your hair.
Friends - winkle you out, when you would rather hide away at home and feel sorry for yourself.
Friends - ignore all 'control freakery'.
Friends - ignore all stroppiness.
Friends - ignore all burbling nonsense.
Friends - send you a card just before an important appointment.
Friends - give you gifts when you don't expect them.
Friends - sit through boring appointments whilst you are being filled up with drugs.
Friends - make you laugh.
Friends - don't mind if you have a hole in your sock.
Friends - pray for you.
Friends - ring you up for a chat.
Friends - make biscuits for you.
Friends - seem to want you to stay around a little longer.
Friends - don't want you to give up.

EXERCISE IS GOOD FOR YOU.

Jenny said that people on Tamoxifen have a tendency to put on weight. I also heard that exercise is very good at de-stressing people. So I have been walking about two miles a day, everyday. It strengthens my bones too. I joined the local library, so that I would have an aim to one of my walks. The librarian was a bit sniffy about my old card. She said it was out of date and she promptly cut it up in front of me, with a bit too much relish, I thought. So I had to re-join and take all sorts of documents, not a passport, oh'no, that wasn't good enough. So I am now "re-activated" and I can take out twelve books at a time.

As I walk along, I talk to myself and my friend "Spike" my inner guide (I will explain him later). I have composed a rhyme which I say in time to my steps.

WALK THE WALK, TALK THE TALK!

My cancer has gone:
My bones are strong:
My (blood) cells are well:
My spine is fine:
My heart is smart:
My brain is the same:
My feet are neat:
My height is right.

I have a pedometer, which is useful for measuring my distance. I have also had a bike ride with Veronica, first time on a bike for thirty years, great fun!

· · · · · ·

I HAD MY OATS.
22/9/2003

I've just finished my second cup of tea and am about to dip into my porridge, when Malcolm said "haven't you got an appointment this morning at 8.30am?"

Blood test for Nottingham next week, I shot out of bed, gave myself a "lick and a promise" don't bother with hair, doesn't make any difference combed or uncombed, hopped around, threw on my clothes, rushed out to the car. Malcolm waved me off in his pyjamas. Completed dressing at the traffic lights, only ten minutes late. I'm running out of places for needles to be stuck into. That's it, I've had enough of needles, appointments etc. etc. etc. nurse very nice and friendly, accepts my apologies, try to compose myself and appear normal. Arrive home and finish porridge which is still warm.

Longest wait ever, at Lincoln Hospital on Friday 19th. One and a half hours to see Dr. E. report backache and explain I'd been bell ringing, hedge cutting and helping to lay paving slabs, so hoped it was that. Did

I want an X-ray, "yes, no, I don't know", "show me where", "that's not your back, that's your side". Check blood test results, -blood count and bone and ask about previous one - liver, calcium and another one. Dr. E gives me the telephone report to keep, so I can see for myself. "So I'm alright", "yes, you know you are!". Another hour to wait for my Zometa, chatted up by several very nice men, who are as bored as I am. No pump for my drip so Chris does it direct, never been done so quickly, all finished in twenty minutes. Nurses short staffed and getting irritable with each other, man has a funny turn across the way, doctor comes. Bad morning I think for everyone, arrive home at 2.00pm. Put blood test results in Red File, may frame it later.

• • • • • •

IMMUNE - SYSTEM CELLS (ORANGE) ATTACKING A CANCER CELL (PINK)

This is a coloured scanning electron micrograph, the killer T-lymphocytes (orange) which are part of the body's immune system, have released a chemical that is killing a cancer cell (pink). As the cell dies, it releases small spheres (in pink).

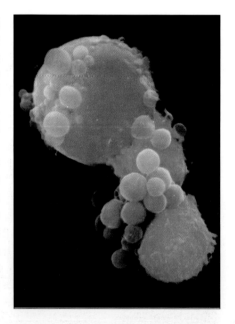

Carina who has just come to live with her mother opposite (separated from her husband, a judge in America) gave me this picture from a magazine. She has a friend who is an oncologist in America; she said my treatment was as good, if not better than in America. Nice to know.

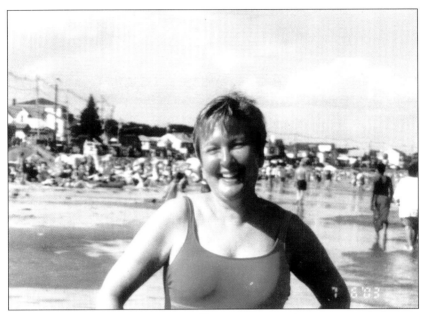

Nancy

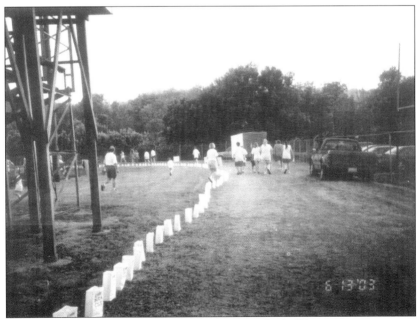

Luminaria at the Harrison County Relay for Life

NANCY
2/10/2003

I have known Nancy over thirty years. We met in Bristol, when I worked in the largest and most awful ESNS School in Europe and she was doing a post graduate American teaching degree, teaching practise. We used to write at Christmas and birthdays. Nancy loved all things English, the history, buildings, accent, everything. I haven't seen Nancy since my time in Bristol, but she doesn't seem to have changed much. Her father was a Lutheran clergyman. She is now married and has two children Carrie and Drew and her husband is Jon.

When she found out about my Breast Cancer, she wrote straight away and did her best to cheer me up in that direct American way. She is very busy teaching English at the local high school and with her two teenage children, but she found time to write letters of encouragement. She also took part in this Relay for Life, Luminaire. I think they light a candle at dusk, for people they know with cancer.

I wasn't sure how I felt when I saw my name there, correctly spelt, all the way over there in America, and as I said to her when I thanked her for her thoughtfulness and her families, I feel I have an affinity now with Nettie and the others.

• • • • • •

KARI
2/10/2003

I have a friend in Norway, Kari, who works, another coincidence, in the cancer hospital in Oslo. I think they only have one hospital, it is very large and she showed us around on one of our visits. The population of Norway is quite small about eight million people. People from the north will not get many visitors. I have known Kari since I was about thirteen years old; we had pen friends to help them learn English. I'm afraid I found Norwegian too hard.

We wrote at Christmas and birthdays too, I had many happy holidays there too, sailing over from Newcastle on the Fred Olsen line - the only person not seasick once on a very bad stormy crossing.

Kari rang me when she found out about my Breast Cancer and talked for ages. I was on my Chemo' so I wasn't very sensible, but I did my best. Next thing a large packet of information came through the post. She works in the laboratory and knows what to look up on the computer. Some of the information frightened the life out of me, not being used to medical jargon and also in denial. They are very cool and collected, Norwegians, matter of fact, and I'm not, I get a bit excited and emotional. I said "I'm in a hole aren't I?" and she said "Yes, you are". Not what I wanted to hear, but she meant well, so I understood her concern.

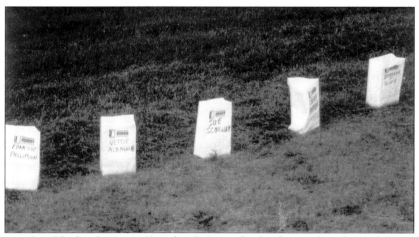

One of the three Luminaries Nancy bought for me. Sue Scouller gets about, doesn't she?

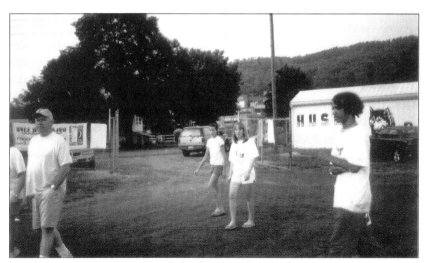

Carrie, Nancy's daughter doing the Relay for Life

CLOSURE
2/10/2003

Check-up at Nottingham, Mr. U. very pleased with his handiwork and himself. I am pleased with the results too. Only fly in the ointment is he is trebling my Thyroxin dose to 75 micrograms now and maybe a 100 mg after the next blood test in six weeks time. I will lose weight and feel better. I was a kilo heavier than before the operation. Sees no reason why I should not join the gym, thinks it can only do me good. Wishes me well and to take care of myself. Nottingham City Hospital certainly took good care of me.

So that's the last visit to Nottingham, I get free prescriptions because I am on Thyroxin, which helps; it was getting expensive with all my pills. I hope there isn't a world shortage of it, but as Sue H. said "not to worry, you will have a cupboard full of spare supplies, like you did at school!" I bequeathed my personal parking cone* to my replacement at school, talking of cupboards. I hope they appreciated it. I said I had had enough of needles last time, but I had my ears pierced on Saturday. The girl who did it told me all about her operation. They didn't want to do it at first, "you will need a doctor's note!" I said I had had more needles stuck into me than I'd had hot dinners and I wasn't moving until they did it!

I kept it in my well stocked cupboard!!

TRUST
6/OCT/2003

What would you do,
If it was you?
What would you say,
If it was your last day?

You wouldn't make a fuss,
Lose your temper, shout and cuss.
You would be calm and brave,
That's how you would behave.

Could I learn to hope and trust?
I should know I must.
Hope and trust, trust and hope, hope and trust I must.

S. Scouller

I must learn to trust Dr. E. when she tells me I am alright and my blood test is alright too. I shall have to prove to them that I am still worth bothering about even though they will not operate and Jenny thinks I am only worth seven years. We shall see!

• • • • • •

POLITENESS

If people ask me,
I always tell them:
"Quite well, thank you, I'm very glad to say".
If people ask me,
I always answer,
"Quite well, thank you, how are you today?"
I always answer,
I always tell them,
If they ask me Politely …. But SOMETIMES
I wish that they wouldn't.

By A. A. Milne.

JIM

"Who is this Jim you keep going to see!

I think Malcolm is a little suspicious of my new found activities with Jim!

I'm in, they have accepted me, and I filled in the disclaimer form and managed to sidestep any mention of cancer. Got them more interested in my operation and thyroid, just mentioned bone strengthening medicine nonchalantly. I don't think they have any idea, wonderful to be just like everyone else.

The gym was Veronica's idea, she is very keen, and showed me around, I did everything she did except running on the treadmill. I did four lengths in the pool, she wouldn't let me do anymore, biked for ten minutes, then ten minutes on the rowing machine. They said light weights would be a good idea to start in a few weeks. I finished off in the steam room, very funny finding the small room full of people and couldn't see any of them. Had a nice conversation with a man about motorbikes. Tried the sauna laid down with another strange man, no conversation this time, too hot. Loved it, must be doing me good and so clean.

Disappointed when I weighed myself, haven't lost any weight at all. My new book recommends an hours exercise, three times a week. I am absolutely determined to get fit, ready for my next blood test. Feel so much better organising myself, doing something for myself.

YEAR 1
5/11/2003

MALCOLM

> **Let me not to the marriage of**
> **true minds admit impediments.**
> **Love is not love which alters when it alteration finds.**

Sonnet 116 - William Shakespeare. 1564-1616

Malcolm is "down in the dumps", hardly surprising really. He has had an awful year. My B.C. and all of that, he lost his job and then his mother died.

Malcolm is highly strung, very clever, sensitive, kind, gentle and quite a lot of other good things. When we married we promised "in sickness and in health" etc. the marriage service is very wise, it knows that life is not going to be easy, we will be tested. As far as I am concerned Malcolm has passed the test. He nursed me when I was very sick, sat through terrible meetings of doom and gloom. He organised the building of the conservatory, so that I could enjoy being in there, painting when it was too cold to be outside. He has done the shopping, cooking, cleaning, washing. He has learnt reflexology to help me, encouraged me to go to the gym. He takes Mum out for days and for a meal and mends things.

He didn't go to his mother's funeral, because I wanted to go with him (2 days travelling, 500 miles) and he didn't want me to face the journey and upset (re-family) and I had to have treatment, he did not want me to miss that session.

He did his own remembrance, we went to the Longland Chantry in Lincoln Cathedral, lit a candle and read though the service at the exact time, the service was held in Inverness. He has donated three trees to the Woodland Trust at Horncastle Carr and we are going to find them, photograph them and put it with the certificate in Memory of his mother.

So he deserves some happy times now and I hope we get it. I feel fine, better than, I have for a long time.

I'm going to let Malcolm check the sell-by dates on my tins in the cupboard. This is one of his favourite jobs, he always finds something out of date and we have a very peculiar time eating up, strange mixtures as I cannot waste them. I told him Captain Scott of the Antartic had tinned food and they opened some recently, which was perfectly alright! Rusty, but alright!

The last paragraph was meant to be light-hearted- I find I have to explain things not everyone has my sense of humour.

No-, how can I begin to repay all the love, kindness and concern, time and goodwill, that has been given to me by Malcolm and everyone else this last year? I can't, but I value every bit of it.

• • • • • •

One step forward two steps back

Lenin 1870-1924

24/11/2003
Just when I thought everything was going well and I wouldn't have anything to report, it all goes "pear shaped".
I've never been in an ambulance before and I don't want to again. Two arrived very quickly. I had started haemorrhaging late Monday night, no pain, no warning just a frightening mess. It stopped and then started again, so we had to do something about it.

A very nice young 'girl' doctor checked me out, glad it wasn't a man, although I noticed she went red in the face fighting the equipment, I'm sure she was more gentle than a man would have been.

The gynaecological ward would not take me, full I suppose, so as it had stopped again I was sent home to see my GP with a letter. After a battle with the receptionist and another session of haemorrhaging, we managed to get an appointment after surgery with my doctor.

He was apologetic and said next time to ring him (if we can get past the receptionist). He gave me pills to stop the bleeding and faxed for a fast track appointment with the gynaecologist consultant for investigations, within two weeks.

It may be a side effect of the Tamoxifen, I have never been great friends with my womb and if it means I can still take Tamoxifen, I will not be sad to part company with it. I'm very disappointed about this setback; I was doing so well, dreadful headache and sick on Wednesday. Malcolm in charge of victuals again, in fact Malcolm in charge of everything at the moment.

> # Human nature seldom walks up to the word 'cancer'.

Rudyard Kipling

9/12/2003

Once again when I am flat on the floor my friends rally round and haul me up again.

Just for a change I am in the Maternity Department and Mr. L. the gynaecologist is examining me. Tells me to put my hands by my side, I'm waving them around again. Not so bad as I expected, no camera, he has given up. I am to have a M.R.I scan to show up the problem and then an internal under anaesthetic. It is the first time I have come close to crying, I feel the tears well up in my eyes, neither of us is under any illusions, I really tried hard to get fit, do as I was told, be positive. Just how much is a person expected to take?

` I wonder, if I see Dr. E. on Friday, what she will say. Irene is sending her mother to be with me that day. She used to be an 'Auntie' at the hospital to help frightened children cope with consultations. I am glad 'Auntie Flo.' is going to be with this frightened child.

Walked to doctor's surgery to find out if my blood test results are back, they are not. Rang Nottingham, surprise, surprise, they are on Mr. U's desk and letter to come. Perhaps a chat with Sarah will cheer me up on Friday.

· · · · · ·

> # Normal service will be resumed as soon as possible.

BBC

14/12/2003

I was so pleased to tell Sarah that I was having my hair cut. She had been very kind about the return of my hair, which had grown back as a curly mop. I said I had lost all my street credibility now; people don't seem to take curly haired people very seriously. I said if I have my hair cut I will lose my strength. I am going to stop being flippant, I said something flippant once before and look what happened.

Sandra asked if I wanted to see Dr. E. this time, I said "yes please". Dr. E. had got Mr. L's letter and asked about the scan and examination. She sat at the side of me and was kind, I looked at her and she looked at me and I felt a little sorry for her all of a sudden, she really looked sorry for what had happened.

I wanted her to know that I didn't blame her and said "I'm sorry about this, it's not your fault, you did your best". She said it wasn't my fault either and I would want to see her at my next Zometa appointment in a month. The results of the tests would be through by then. I have another specialist nurse called Heather, spoke to her on the telephone. I'm going to ask her why I'm having a chest X-ray.

· · · · · ·

MRI MAGNETIC RESONANCE IMAGING
19/12/2003

High quality images of the internal parts of the body without the use of X-rays. It uses a large powerful magnet and radio waves.

"Ground Control to Major Tom, …Ground Control to Major Tom". "Put your space suit on". "Are you alright, loud voice coming, this one for seven minutes". I'm pushed into a large polo mint shaped machine; headphones clamped to my ears and panic button and lead grasped in my hand. They put Classic FM on the radio, but it didn't drown out the noise, a bit like a noisy two stroke engine that vibrated a lot. About six sessions of five or six minutes each and different noises. Now they grab my arm to put in a dye, I protest, "I'm having a blood test at 4pm". "Oh, it will be gone by then". Oh, well why should I worry if they think I have blue blood.

For once I don't mind being helped by two young men who hauled me upright, one carried my basket of clothes back to the changing room for me and tried to be helpful, said they had taken eighty photo's and shook hands with me- I'm worried now, why is he being so nice to me. "When are you seeing your doctor?". I say "which one!" Chest X-ray for pre-op. checks. Pre-op checks Christmas Eve.

70

Nil desperandum - Never despair

Horace 65-8 BC.

Britain - The land of embarrassment and breakfast

Julian Barnes

• • • • • •

31/12/2003
HYSTEROSCOPY

My inspection operation is on New Years Eve. I have had pre-op test and explanations. They are going to do unspeakable things to my bladder and womb. "Don't worry if they make a hole in either, they will repair it" - that's alright then. They are all being very nice to me despite my dejected attitude. I say I don't want to play hospitals anymore; I want to play airlines or any new game. How am I going to face the results, no Beth this time?

• • • • • •

TEST RESULTS
9/1/2004

The "sword of Damodes" is hanging by a thread.
Hanging there, precariously above my head.

Supported, uncertain, by a hair.
How long will it, can it, be there?

S. Scouller

71

Dr. E. was sure the histology results would be back, but they were not back. Mr. L. writes his reports in red ink and although neat, she finds them hard to read (a ploy to find out what I know?) I did my best to recall what he had said post op. She said she would ring up and get the results. I said I didn't want to know. We had another battle of wills. I said I knew I had to know but I didn't want to know. I asked about my last blood test, I went through everything on the form, kidney liver function, bone, full blood count all ok a change of tablet was mentioned, other than Tamoxifen. No results, more tests needed, I thought on me, but Malcolm thinks on the biopsy.

A boy of twenty was in the waiting room one Friday, with his parents. He was quietly being sick into one of those paper bowls, people looking sideways at him. He has brain cancer. I had better stop feeling sorry for myself.

Good news chest X-ray clear, bad news cancer is in the cervix and lining of the womb. Specialist nurse Heather tells me over the phone at my request. I say I'm pleased Dr. E. didn't tell me, because she was Dr. 'Bad News' before and it had taken me nearly a year to get over that. She can be Dr. 'Good News' now with treatment for me.

Jenny rang with sympathy, I think it is best if I get over my resentment of her. I decide to ask for a talk and maybe give her an idea of the questions before hand to save time.

I retire to bed to lick my wounds, Sue H and Veronica alarmed to hear this. I keep being sick and feel very sorry for myself. I know I have to come out and face it. Pep talk from V! AM phone call "are you out of bed?" "YES".

JENNY (1ST RESERVE)
30/1/2004

> **"Now this is not the end. It is not even the beginning of the end. But it is, perhaps, the end of the beginning".**

Winston Churchhill. 1874-1965

I called for help, I needed it, I decided to give Jenny a chance to shine and admit I needed help. I hoped to get rid of my resentment of previous conversations. She had always acted quickly on my behalf before with admin requests and organised things, it was just the personal bit, I couldn't get behind the eyes.

To my surprise she suggested a home visit. This made it much easier for me, I could relax and Malcolm could be there. I kept to my points, rambled off the point at times and there was a lot of "I wants". I tried to explain how I felt and I hoped she understood, I risked telling her things I would normally only share with close friends, for fear of being thought 'potty', but I wanted her to join my team and use her skills and expertise to help me.

I managed to do the whole talk without mentioning Beth, when just at the end Malcolm asked how she was, I was a little cross, because it was Jenny's session, I didn't want to annoy her. She said she was nearly better and hoping to come back at Easter, she said she would want to know she had been looking after her patients! I said I had better behave and 'buck-up'!! God does answer prayers doesn't he?

BETH'S BETTER
27/1/2004

I must have got it right.
I asked most every night.

So many things to say.
I did not know the way.

To keep it to the gist,
I had a little list.

I sometimes fell asleep,
Too tired to even weep.

It's 'GOODNEWS' day today,
And all I did was pray.

S. S

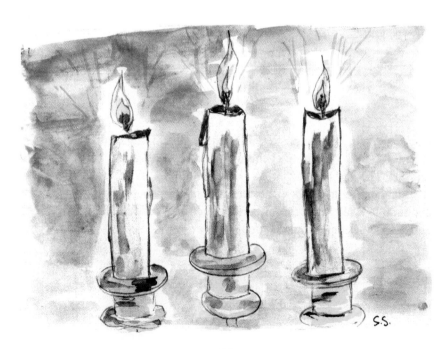

RADIOTHERAPY
'DR. E. SAID I AM WORTH IT!'

Everything seems so much easier when you have done it all before. I had queried rectum on the Activity sheet, I thought it was pelvis. Jenny said someone had pressed the wrong code button and I was quite right to ask about it. I put my jogging bottoms on for ease of dressing etc. and sport three new tattoos. I said don't put all my tattoos in a line or I will fall apart at the perforations! Then I was told I had to see Dr. E. to sign the consent form. Panic, me in my sloppy trousers, I hadn't expected that.

Dr. E. sat at the side of me and we went thro' the form, said I was glad she was in charge --- "because you would have it all at once", "yes and in a complete muddle". I said I hoped it worked or I would be up the creek without a paddle. "You have three paddles, Radiotherapy, Chemo and Arimidex". I suddenly found I was inundated with paddles in my canoe in my imagination. She said I was getting the treatment because I was worth it. I didn't know how to respond but I thought it was a very nice thing to say. She said it again as I went out of the door. She is obviously doing her best for me. We had a chat about overseas staff "I am from overseas" and the need for interpreters, "they say I have an accent still". I said I had an accent and the overseas staff probably spoke better English than I did. I think she would like to talk about where she comes from. I am getting better at consultations, so I may ask her which hot country one day when she is not busy

Saw Sarah on Friday morning for my Zometa. Jill said as I came thro' the door "have you been here all night?" I managed a reply, "yes thought it would save time". Had a good chat with Sarah, didn't mention my setback. Sandra, ward clerk is very nice to me, calls me by my christian name and is very helpful.

I shall have to think up some new themes to pass the time every appointment. We didn't do Dr. Who. I made Jenny laugh, telling her about the klingons and how the boss, Liz, was not too pleased at being designated one. I also made her laugh about the pain down my face after my thyroid operation and how I was going to ask for pain killers, when I discovered it was the elastic band rubbing on my ear, from the oxygen mask!

Rather like the chair I always use when I go to the clinic. Front of house, I am near both doors to hear my name and I get nice "hellos" and smiles from people coming and going. I wonder if they think I am the usherette or something. I have a wonder round, they have got used to that too!

• • • • • •

WAITING
17/2/2004

Always the same,
Whenever they call her name,
Where is Sue?
She's gone to the loo!

Always much to do,
And where was Sue?
No time to stop and stare,
She was never there.

It will always be the same,
She will listen for her name,
Where will you be Sue?
"Here and there and everywhere,
I'll be somewhere new….with you".

S.Scouller

• • • • • •

REMEMBER
FOR JANE
18/2/2004

Remember happy days, those lazy lazy summer days.
The sun shines warm, the insects hum,
Time suspended, time for fun.

A stream to ford, to splash and paddle,
A conversation with the cattle.

Trees to climb, rooks a huddle,
A great big enormous puddle.

Remember brown Auturnal days,
The wet look leaves,
Free fruit on the trees.
Natures cycle of decay.

Remmember Winters icy slide,
How, on frosty nights I loved to hear
Ancient bells sound crisp and clear.

Remember sticky buds, catkins and brave
Bright flowers of Spring.
Fledglings wobbling on the wing.

Will you remember all these to see?
Will you remember me?

S. Scouller

• • • • • •

CONFESSION
19/2/2004

I think I better come clean,
I'm not the person I seem.

I've a sercet I've tried to keep,
Did I talk of it… not a peep.

Shall I now confess to you,
These things I cannot do!

Algebra, fractions, geometry too,
Quadratic equations and calculus, phew!

S. Scouller

MY GUARDIAN ANGEL

20/2/2004

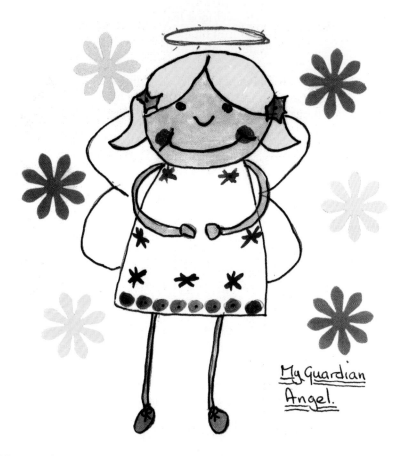

My Guardian Angel.

I have a tiny Angel; she lives in my pocket, that's where she has her fun, because God is so busy, with far too much to do. He said that what she has to do is keep watch over me. Then he tucked her in my pocket, Blessing me with Angel care, and she promised to stay right there! So, if ever I am lonely and my hearts in need of love, I just touch her in my pocket and she will give me love from above.

GOD BLESS FROM MY GUARDIAN ANGEL.

THE JOURNEY
21/2/2004

Hope said to Comfort:-
"We must follow the light, if we follow the light,
We will be alright".
Comfort said to Hope:-
"We have done our best, our very best, we will soon have rest".
Doubt said to Dispair:-
"Our situations very dire, we're in a mire a deep, dark mire".
Despair said to Doubt:-
"I'm giving-up and giving-in, I'm sure we cannot win".
Wisdom said to Lost:-
"Help willingly is given, you only have
To ask, you only have to ask, for help along the way".
Lost said to Wisdom:-
"Now I reject my pride, my prickly pride, let friends and God be on my
side".

S. Scouller.

With acknowledgements to John Bunyan.

ARIMIDEX
PADDLE NUMBER ONE
28/2/2004

Talking to Dr. W. my GP I discover that Arimidex, the pills Dr. E. has replaced my Tamoxifen with, are very expensive, about £100 for a months supply, compared with £7.50p for Tamoxifen. I am shocked; he said I wasn't to feel guilty. I must do well now; Beth said they spent "megabucks".

• • • • • •

SUE IN HER CANOE
PADDLE NUMBER TWO
1/3/2004

Dr. E. did warn me it wouldn't be as easy as before. By the end of the second week I'm feeling the side-effects. Found a new friend, a man who makes model railways. He seems very perky, havn't asked what's wrong with him, we walk to the main entrance together to get our tickets stamped.

Have a check due with Dr. E. on Friday after treatment. Dr. E. doesn't finish her ward rounds until about 9.30am so I know I'll have to wait.

'Leading Lady' Sandra takes me under her wing as soon as I appear in the main waiting room. She organises a mug of tea for me from Ingham Ward, and fends off a member of staff giving me 'duff' information about when I will be seen. I am very grateful; I put drops of ginger essence on my biscuits to stop the nausea, which starts straight away. There is another side-effect which I will not share with you!

Dr. E. seems pleased and I say I think something is working because the symptoms have eased. She asks if I would like to have my Zometa now, instead of next Friday when it is due. I agree and she organises it with Ingham Ward, she knows I'll be on my knees by them!

• • • • • •

BED
2/3/2004

"Have you any idea, of the fear, in my head Bed?"
"As you stand there four square".

"Lie down on the bed", she said,
Such a simple request.
Said the bed, "be my gueat".

I'm completely supine
Everything should be fine
So what's the unease?
Explain to me please.

Said the Bed, "Relax!
Lie down like a lamb,
And forget the exam,
Horizontal is best,
When you're needing a rest".

"Our talk has been helpful", I said to the bed,
"I think I will manage it now without dread".

S. Scouller

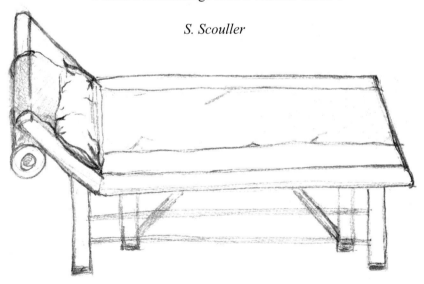

MR THING
6/3/2004

There is this 'Thing'.
He sits on my shoulder
And is annoying me,
What could it be?

He will not go away
He sits there all the day
And he is a nuisance.
I call him Mr. Thing.

He whispers in my ear
When I am feeling down
"You really ought to know
It's nearly time to go".

"Mr. Thing, please go away
I want to live just one more day".
Besides I want to be the one to say
I'll not be told by anything.

S. Scouller.

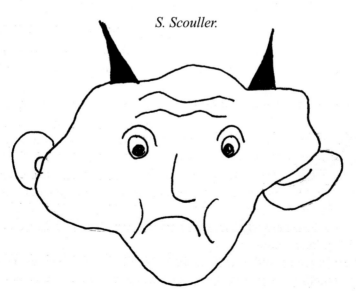

He who can, does. He who cannot, teaches.

George Bernard Shaw

7/3/2004

Before I trained to teach in a Special School, I worked a year as a 'dogsbody' at the Special School in Louth.

The first job I learnt was to make the tea to everyones liking. I then went from class to class helping and learning. I started with the nursery and worked my way thro' to 'children' who were bigger than me in age and size.

Everything was fine until the teacher left the room and what appeared to be a roomful of little angels turned instantly into a room of little devils.

I soon realised that all the preparation, equipment, theory was as naught compared to the teachers character and personality. Nothing could or would be done if there wasn't that invisible bond between the teacher and class. How to get that intangible bond? The children were certainly not going to give their trust, respect or friendship to anyone they hadn't thoroughly vetted first and why should they.

So it was trial by fire, hell and high water, you name it they did it. If you were still there and still loved them despite their drawbacks and they had plenty of those and were not put off by the poor hand dealt to them in looks and brain power, then they might accept you into their world. They would of course keep you continually up to the mark more efficiently than any OFSTED inspection, but they would open up and let you feel honoured to be one of them.

They would show thus in little ways, like the time Charlie brought me a big bunch of tulips for my desk, which I proudly displayed. I noticed on the way home that tulips of the same colour seemed to have disappeared from the garden under the Head's window.

Or when Paul, whose father was a dustman, brought me exciting presents of an old clock and broken bits of electrical equipment recycled from the dustbins.

They would generously share their sweets, which were delicious once the fluff had been removed.

I of course lived in the stock cupboard and one very good test was to give me something, a responsibility, such as looking after a precious doll from their life support system (school bag), knowing, if it was Friday, I would have to look after it until Monday morning.

We took them in the summer holidays for a weeks stay at the Leicester Boys Home, Mablethorpe. It was a bit spartan, but the sun shone and sand and sea was good fun. Josie took a shine to me, she was one of the senior girls, square shaped and solid. She frequently had tantrums and would bang her head on the wall screaming defiance. I called her 'Twinkle Toes' which caught her imagination, she was light on her feet, but that was all. Anyway she insisted upon walking with me, sitting with me and would not go to sleep at night until I had told her a story and kissed her goodnight.

She liked to paddle in the sea, when the water was around her waist I was sent to retrieve her, as if she would take any notice of me! Everyone was watching me from the safety of sand dunes, waiting for the expected tantrum. I knew Josie liked her tummy more than even paddling. I suggested she came in and have her dinner; it was her favourite (I'd talk my way out of that one later). A grunt was the answer to that, they were all watching, Josie had won, I was useless. One last try "I shall be sad not to sit next to you at dinner Twinkle Toes". I turned and walked back to the dunes and there she was, wet up to her arms, walking back with me. As a special treat Josie sat next to me at the cinema that evening. I can't remember what the film was, I hardly heard the soundtrack, Josie had fallen asleep, she was contently snoring loudly beside me. I ignored all the looks and went to sleep too, my hand firmly gripped in Josie's. I wasn't going anywhere.

I'm not what you would call a tights person. I was never impressed with stockings or got to grips with tights. They either tied my knees together or needed constantly hitching up. So I had genuine sympathy with Susan when she flushed her new bra down the school lavatory blocking the drains. Susan's father had donkeys on the beach at Mablethorpe. I mean really, when a girl is used to freedom, who wants to be trussed up with a bra.

Some of the children were seasonal, from travelling families. Benjamin was small with shiny chestnut brown eyes and a permanent smile. Nothing ever dented Benjamin's self-confidence and good humour. He didn't even mind when we got changed for P.E. and his socks stayed vertical like miniature Wellington boots. Superior socks, that's what he had and positive thinking.

So I went off to college well armed with practical experience to train in Leeds. From the sublime to the ridiculus, inner city tough children. Sometimes it wasn't the children who were difficult, it was the staff. On teaching practise if you dared to sit in the wrong chair in the staff room or if you got something right, they didn't like you. I found main stream teachers harsher on me than E.S.N teachers.

I had great respect for the teachers of East End Park School. The headmistress locked the main school door at 9.00am and watched thro' her office window for any irate parents storming across the playground.

We did old fashioned 'drill' in the playground for P.E. and they loved it. We also did that new fangled music and movement. The teacher stood in the middle of the hall, window pole in her hand, and whacked any dilatory interpretation of the music. Be a butterfly…"whack", now gentle fairy footsteps…"whack". If only the lady on the radio could see how we jumped around.

We had a session at the local baths once a week. There were a lot of uncleared bomb sites still in the early '60s and we picked our way across these and thro' the allotments in single file. The West Indian children balancing the kit on their heads, their deportment already much better than mine.

My favourite time was assembly. I thought it was a good idea to play classical music to the children to calm them down and hopefully open their ears to other kinds of culture. The children were very enthusiastic, I couldn't believe how carefully all these tough children listened to the William Tell Overture. Hardly a word spoken, intense concentration. I soon found out why, they were waiting for the part when it sounds as though the cavalry has arrived. Not only that, they all started to ride their chairs with gusto. It was bedlam.

I enjoyed living in Leeds, we had no money, were freezing cold most of the time but the people made it interesting and worthwhile. Always ready to help with directions, "turn left at Batty's brush factory love". The magnificent buildings, I always wondered why there was a smell of soap at the back of the Town Hall. I imagined someone having a bath in the cellar.

The Craven Dairy shops, useful for a bap at lunch time. These ranged from expensive - roast beef/pork down to spam. It was my ambition to buy a roast beef bap one day.

There was always something going on. I remember I went to the University Union just to post a letter and came out with 50 Rag mags to sell. I sat outside Marks & Spencer in Briggate and sold them all, walked back home, met some friends and went to the cinema, put my tin of money under the seat and promptly kicked it over in a quiet bit. It rolled all the way down to the front me searching in the dark, getting shushed and told off.

Only to arrive back and find I had been reported missing to the police.

My friend reasoned that as I had missed my tea, I must have been abducted (she was very keen on the White Slavery theory). I had to ring the police and say "you know that girl reported missing, well she's not missing anymore". I didn't want them to know it was me ringing, I was very embarrassed. "Thank you for telling us and what's your name and who are you?". Oh dear.

We went out on Friday and Saturday nights, I had one dress and Catherine had one dress, so we alternated each week. We thought we were the 'Bee knees'! The way to our hearts being central heating and a good plate of food, and we still played hard to get.

Excitement one night when we had a breakin, we missed all the fun. The police searched each room and under our beds for the intruder. Catherine and I slept thro' it all, we were so cross. Goodness knows what they thought of us in our bed kit, jumpers bed socks etc.

We learnt the medical aspects of our job; part of this was to visit Meanwood Hospital in Leeds and Westwood Hospital in Bradford. There I saw things that were shocking but true, things I have never forgotten.

· · · · · ·

I WONDER
1/04/2004

Does a tumour have humour,
Is it really a shy, nice guy?

Is it just misunderstood,
And would prefer to be good?

Is it only a cell,
Trying hard to rebel?

Is it making sure, I'll not ignore,
My body anymore?

S. Scouller

CHECK-UP
2/4/2004

Jenny organises my mammogram, before my Zometa appointment. I manage to sketch the dreaded bed, after a chat with Sandra, she is going to Turkey and her little boy is not keen on having his injections. Sandra is concerned about this and she is going to have hers at the same time. I have sympathy with her boy.

I can hear Dr. E. ringing up about me, my name and date of birth. The consulting room is starting to become a problem. I get up and have a good look around. I am going to examine the electrical equipment (no touching!). I still don't know what it is used for, I turn around and there is Dr. E. watching me, I feel like a naughty child. She explains what it is for, I would like to talk more about it, but I feel I am wasting her time.

I report my sickness and nausea and also lumps in my neck. Dr. E. feels it and says nothing; I say can you feel it, yes she can and smacks my hand for touching it again. She says, "it will know I know it is there and get bigger" and not to touch it. I can see the logic. She organises another blood test for Liver, CEA and CA153 to be done on Ingham Ward.

I get the 'third degree' on Ingham Ward when I'm given my Zometa. A nurse, I have only had once before, when she forgot to give me my Zometa after Chemo', so I had to have two injections, asked question after question about my setback in a very unfriendly way. I began to feel I had made a fuss about nothing until I remembered the op. and radiotherapy. I can feel my back going up; I must not lose my temper. Why doesn't she explain what it is all about, what is the problem?

Sickness gets so bad that I am hardly eating or sleeping. Malcolm rings Jenny and speaks to her, he is so worried. I have lost three pounds this week. I look in the mirror haunted eyes and hollow cheeks look back at me. Someone says I look well, I deel like 'death warmed up' despondent. Must organise the 'Enduring power of attorney' for Malcolm at the solicitors, think about hymns.

87

JANE'S POEM FOR ME.
15/4/2004

You spoke of Nature's beauty that each season brings anew
You asked if, at some future time, I might remember you.

You spoke of Nature's beauty - how you hold each season dear,
With contrasts in the colours of the turning of the year.

You care about such simple things as lichen on the wall,
Or snowdrops on a shady bank, the barn owl's twilight call.

You spoke of how, in Summertime, to you the earth seems blessed
As apples ripen on the trees and fledglings fly the nest.

The daisies twinkling in the grass, the blue of August skies,
Such simple beauty always finds the blessing of your eyes.

You feel the warmth in Autumn-time where others see the cold
As colours paint the trees in vivid red and burning gold

You talked of chiming church bells ringing clear in Wintr'ry dawn,
Of ice on frozen cobwebs and bright frost upon the lawn.

You talked about the things you loved, the animals, the birds.
You spoke of Nature's beauty, and you painted it with words.

You asked if I'd remember you in times to come, and yet -
You are Nature's beauty. So, how can I forget?

Jane Clark

88

PADDLE NUMBER THREE.
SUE IN HER CANOE.
28/4/2004

'Non omnis moriar'

Odeo. - Horace 65-8 BC

I think Dr. E. had hoped that the Arimidex would have had time to start working and would have held things at bay for longer. However there is no denying the liver blood test result. She goes straight into action, chest X-ray results for Friday and organises the Chemo (Yew Tree) which she had been keeping in reserve.

So paddle number three comes winging thro' the air, nearly hitting me on the head, to help me paddle my canoe. I must get organised, I have been going round in circles. I take the news better, getting used to it, although, I just knew there was something wrong. I listened to my body that time. I managed the consultation even better, Malcolm was there, he was removed to sit on the bed so Dr. E. could sit at my side and go thro' the consent form.

She must have been tired, a long working week, yet she gave me a friendly dig in the ribs with her elbow, was kind about my hair loss, we had a joke about that, and I told her (she mentioned men coping with this and then we looked at Malcolm. I had loved Malcolm with hair and I love him without hair. It is what's underneath that is important. She agreed, quite a nice moment, Malcolm cheered up! I said he was going to get a medal for looking after me so well. I was 'souped' up on steroids again, so it was quite lively, I said I thought it had got into my brain and she said it was not in my brain, thank goodness.

Sarah gave me my first dose; I'm having one a week for eighteen weeks. She went thro' the do's and don'ts again, ring up the ward if I get a temperature; she tactfully pointed out the advice on sex. I said I was all for it and wasn't that something coal is delivered in, in Scotland!

Have to ring the Medilink Doctor on Monday night because I have a temperature. More antibiotics. Go to my own GP for 'Happy Pills'.

Dr. E. has one more paddle a smart pill Xeloda, which we talk about. I'm not sure if it is Chemo' or not. She said the Docetaxel (Yew Tree) chemo' is more expensive and works quicker and I'm worth it again. I do like it every time she says that. She gave me a pat on the back and was very friendly, I said I wanted them to give me the Chemo' even if I crawled in on my hands and knees.

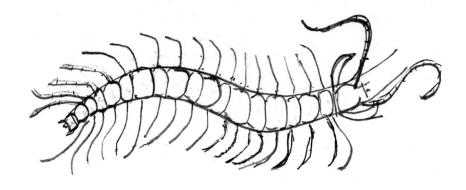

CENTIPEDE
28/4/2004

Centipede, centipede
I think your feet
Are rather neat.

Do you play a tune with a spoon,
Get in a muddle when you juggle
On street corners?

Centipede, centipede
Do you need,
A long seat,
For your feet?
When you are tired.

S. Scouller

NOTES WRITTEN BY SUE
IN HER LAST WEEK, RECORDED
AS WRITTEN.

The meeting made me upset and I was very sick. I mustn't swallow, thank goodness. I think I was cornered. She set up catch Sue plan. Malcolm thinks they are doing a "child study on me".

MONDAY

Tuesday AM. Sue, I saw pink plastic string around the lampshade and bulb. Checked then didn't.

The D. N. said if you crush ice lollies and take them with a spoon, they don't have to be swallowed to get absorbed. So I tried it this A.M and got rid of that much this morning. This was good because I can't take pills, except liquid med. Messy eating

I've got tummy ache, which pill stops this and tummy ache or will I have to sit on a bucket all night.

An hour late, all excuses, hosp? No. Left one worse, Sarah blister expert called; to dress it (L) one wouldn't touch (R) leg. Locum. Leg burst about 10am and dressed R leg. (Has all proper equipment).

Sarah put pressure on me (little chat) to have Dis' Nur. , 'no thanks', this morning decide the references to Malcolm and managing perhaps should agree.

Dis Nurse arranged for Sunday but she came AM. Explained my work to 3 practise Dis NURSES.

They had got this organised they used Sarah, because they (knew) I would not give in and they used Malcolm, saying he needed respite care. They knew I would not give in, lots of droopy faces.

Dr. E had reserved a bed. They knew I would do it for Malcolm. I said no, and then I thought about it long and hard. They made me feel I was being hard to Malcolm. They really put pressure on me for my obstinacy. Had double vision, jerking and I was sick. Dr. E. has made a big mistake, she thinks I am like everyone else. This hurt, Dr. E's pride, I said I wasn't blaming, anyone. They know they have to come up with a good reason

they know they will not pull the wool over my eyes. They knew there would be trouble, she had everyone primed. Sandra, Betty, Ann-Marie, Jill. Long faces everyone, it was last appointment. They didn't know, we had I kept them dry and I had kept of them.....
   I had flashing just then, funny vision, starbursts,

Notes written by Sue, to describe photographs I had taken in the garden to show her how it was looking, as she had not been able to go outside, but only to look out of the window

Used to be at gate post never grew.
Top of Malcolm's tripod granddad's rose cutting used to be at back on post.
Cistus,
Hanging Baskets,
roses from Granddad's cuttings, light pink
Cistus,
Hebe looking towards side entrance near weather instruments and wheelie bin.
Granddad's light pink rose from cutting.
Small white rose over arbour, Rambling Rector.
Two of granddad's roses from cuttings at side of conservatory.
New fruit trees at bottom.
New garden by side of seat.
Cuttings grown in tubs.
Apple or pear trees.
Bottom of garden.
Arbour from the side.
Himalayan broom yellow, nice scent very expensive.
Malcolm's tripod.
Malcolm steps.
Veronica's lily (white).
Irene and Angela's roses and Veronica's lily (white)
Sorry just taken morphine.
I keep getting tapped on the head and called Angel and then fall.
Fall asleep from morphine.

The yellow wet wipes do not flush, you have to put them in the bin.

NOT ORANGE.
Are you sure it's LINCOLN Hosp not LOUTH? Hosp.

THE LAST WEEKS BY MALCOLM

The following diary was written after Sue's death and is not necessarily an exact description of her last few weeks, some details are out of sequence, but it does not change the story.

FRIDAY 30/4/2004
Sue had her second dose of Docetaxel chemo' and monthly Zometa.

SATURDAY 1/5/2004
I went shopping at Staples and B&Q while Sue rested.

SUNDAY 2/5/2004
Another quiet day, Sue is getting a sore mouth.

MONDAY 3/5/2004
Sue's mouth is very sore and she is finding eating food very difficult, soups, jelly, etc. only. I went to the chemist and bought a tube of mouth ulcer cream. Soothes for a while.

TUESDAY 4/5/2004
Sue has very sore mouth with ulcers. I decide next day we must do something about it, as she is already on antibiotics for her raised temperature, which started after her first Docetaxel chemo'.

WEDNESDAY 5/5/2004
Took Sue to the doctor with very bad mouth, large ulcers, and the doctor takes one look and says he will not do anything. Instead rings Ingham Ward, who say go home and we will contact you. Drive home, find message on answer machine from ward nurse. Ring back and they say we should see Dr. E. in her clinic in the out-patient department as soon as possible, but do not rush up, also they will admit her to Wragby Ward for a few days. We pack a bag for Susie with washing kit, spare clothes, nightdresses, slippers, radio etc.

Proceed to Lincoln County hospital, park near as possible to out-patients, and go into clinic. We do not have to wait long, as we are called through to see Dr. E. very quickly. She is a little surprised at the extent of the ulcers, only seen one bad case before. She organises a blood test and arranges admission to Wragby Ward for Sue. So off we go to blood clinic, we wait awhile as it's busy at that time of day. Then we proceed to the ward which is a long way off on the floor above the Chemo' out-patients department.

On arrival we are directed to the Day Room as no bed is available at the moment. Lots of people are waiting for a bed for their chemo'. Sue very tired and she falls asleep, meantime I realise Pat from my old work place is there doing a puzzle while waiting to be discharged. She had Breast Cancer many years ago and now has further problems. We chat about this and that while waiting for a very long time, Sue is in the loo feeling sick when we are eventually called to a bed. A nurse comes and takes all Sue's details, Sue can't talk much so I have to fill in some of the details. Then we settle down to await the doctor, who is very busy as she is a locum, and has all the regular chemo' patients to see so they can get started. Apparently one doctor has left and the other is on holiday, just our luck to strike a good day!

Eventually she arrives and we go through everything again, she looks at Sue's mouth and eventually prescribes medicine for thrush and a drip for liquid. They still think she can swallow and try giving her painkillers by mouth, but not with too much success unfortunately. Sue is unhappy with one senior staff nurse who she christens 'Matron' for her attitude, yes poor old Sue took 'offence' and it was a long time before she got over her. I went home and did some jobs returning in the evening for another visit. Pat is in the next bed, although she has gone home after bad news we think.

THURSDAY 6/5/2004

Sue H. visits and organises mouth wash swabs and liquids. Sue arranges everything on her meal table so it is all within reach. Cups of Aspirin mouth wash, clean water, folded paper towels, sick bowl, swabs, dissolved solpadols etc. Very well organised and she would get annoyed if you moved anything**. She was not eating or drinking so she was on a saline drip, but we did manage to organise Dia-morphine injections as she was not able to swallow the solpadols.

** My Mum would keep her things in a certain order on the table next to her chair at home.

SATURDAY 8/5/2004

Visited Sue.

SUNDAY 9/5/2004
Visited Sue, she was hoping to come home tomorrow.

MONDAY 10/5/2004
As well as me, Sue H., Veronica and others have been to see Sue, so she has had plenty of visitors. Too many in fact, as she has to write things down to communicate with people.

Sue is in a female only ward with six beds, most of the ladies are in for chemo' sessions that can't be done in the day ward. Staff all very friendly and kind, for ever dashing about sorting out bleeping chemo' delivery machines, as they can block at the smallest amount of arm waving sometimes. Although they are on wheels and do manage to travel very well; I have even seem people walking round the hospital grounds with them.

I don't remember days exactly, but Sue had a visit from Dr. E. during ward rounds, who asks another doctor to have a look at her mouth. He comes while I am there and changes the diagnosis to 'Hepes' and suggests a different medicine. (So that's anti-bacterial and anti-fungus medicines being tried)

TUESDAY 11/5/2004
Go to see Sue, only to find she has been moved to the 'broom cupboard', well that's what we called it. Actually it's a room at the end of a corridor with en-suite shower, loo and basin. View is not so good, only a courtyard, whereas from the other ward you could see the prison. We, I think are supposed to wear gloves and aprons so as not to become infected, but it's more important for the staff not to pass it onto other patients. At least Sue can have a shower with a bit of help from the staff and loo is empty except when I am in there. The TV has no remote control so she can't use it unless she gets out of bed.

WEDNESDAY 12/5/2004 TO FRIDAY 14/5/2004
No recall of details other than visiting Sue everyday.

On Friday Sue asks Dr. E. to let her go home on Monday, its yes provided in the meantime she eats bananas, milk and at least three Build-up drinks a day.

SATURDAY 15/5/2004
Sue has been managing to drink Build-up drinks and glasses of milk and

eat ice cream and bananas, so she's hoping to come home on Monday. Over the weekend Dr. Several is back as a locum, and we have a couple of long chats with him, which helps ease Sue's unhappiness with his previous remarks at the clinic.

SUNDAY 16/5/2004

Dr. Several detects a low blood potassium level and Sue goes back on a drip to help correct this problem. Her legs have also become very swollen, but nobody to me appears concerned about the problem.

Maybe I just don't ask the right person, the right questions. All along I have felt a big lack of communication with the staff. I had expected them to volunteer as much detail as possible, approaching me not waiting to be asked. My problem is that if you don't know what's wrong how can you ask questions? I needed a daily briefing on Sue's progress, but finding anybody who could answer questions was difficult. We found the same in Inverness when my Mum was in hospital, it was nothing like the telly programmes where relatives always seem to be getting briefings from doctors. If the doctors don't brief the relatives I suppose the audience would never know what was going on!

MONDAY 17/5/2004

Sue comes home. She has amassed so much extra stuff I have to make three journeys to the car to take clothes, extra Build-up drinks, flowers in vases, etc. on a very hot day. Find wheel chair and wheel Sue out to the car as she is very weak on her legs which are very swollen with water retention. On the way we say thank you and goodbyes to some of the staff. Getting the wheel chair across to the car is interesting, when trying to ride over the bumps and slopes put on the pavement edges at crossing points for blind people. We get stuck on the other side by a mere little rise in the kerb, these wheel chairs are fine on flat floors, but not much use outside. Only other way was to bring the car to the main entrance, but it is very busy with ambulances and taxis and is crowded with smokers, patients as well as staff. It's more like the entrance to a pub bar than a hospital. Could have been better designed; but the architect maybe has never been in a wheel chair or understood just how much space is required outside the entrance for dropping off and picking up patients.

Reminds me of all those supermarket car parks with roads running right pass the entrance, so everybody coming and going (with trolleys, kids etc.) has to walk across the path of departing cars. It's probably one

96

of these draft ideas, to do with access for ambulances or fire engines, but their visits are so rare, the customer's safety should be paramount. Once again it's down to the designers and planners not having a clue about how these buildings are going to be used on a daily basis. Roll on the day when architects are trained to design practical solutions, to life's difficulties. Any body fancy cleaning (dusting) the new Scottish Parliament Chamber?

TUESDAY 18/5/2004

Let battle commence! Sue had promised me that when she came out of hospital she would start eating again! However she is really only eating Build-up drinks and I am finding it very difficult to get her to eat solid foods. I did have great success with my milkshakes, made in the liquidiser, which we normally only use for making Yorkshire Pudding mixture. They had banana, milk, raspberry juice, ice-cream and sometimes orange and kiwi fruit in them to boost her potassium levels.

MONDAY 24/5/2004

Sue has an appointment with Dr. E. to see if she is well enough to continue with the Docetaxel chemo' treatment. Dr. E. prescribes potassium tablets for her low potassium levels and water tablets for her legs. She is happy to try the Docetaxel again as she is sure the mouth ulcers will not return, as they are now convinced it was a bacteria connected to her cold sores, that she probably got years ago from some charming child she taught. These things are pretty common which usually don't bother most healthy people, but during chemo' you are very vulnerable to such infections.

We are sent to X-ray department for another chest X-ray, Sue goes in a wheelchair which I push through long hospital corridors. On the way a very nice porter passes on his tips on how best to steer the wheelchair to keep it in a straight line and lessen the amount of weaving about the corridor. On arrival we are asked to wait, seems very quiet as it's nearly lunchtime, but then I see a notice saying there is a two hour wait. On enquiry it's confirmed as one/two hours. Return to Sue and pass on bad news, I decide to go and buy a Mars bar and bottle of milk. We tried a drink of water earlier to pass the time. We are entertained by our nearest patients; one is obviously from prison as she is chained to two guards. A family across the way has to dash to accident and emergency as another family member is reported to have been admitted. Poor Sue is getting very tired and bored; we try the magazines for the third time, not much to choose from, but can't really concentrate on the articles.

Suddenly we are called to the next station and we are directed to a cubicle were Sue has to change; she is then called to the X-ray room. I push the wheelchair out of cubicle expecting the nurse to take over, but not so, I dash back for Sue's handbag, then they take over thank goodness. After waiting for the film, which I try unsuccessfully to place in holder on chair, it's too big for the holder, we return to the clinic Sue holding the film envelope. On the way over we were allowed out via the back door of the clinic; on return however I have to go outside and along a short stretch of pavement to get to the main entrance to the clinic. Sounds simple does it not? Well not really, as the pavement slopes away from the building towards the road and I have great difficulty in either not ending up in the road or hitting the wall. We arrive in the clinic, to be greeted by concerned faces as to where have we been? They were so concerned they had rung the X-ray department to enquire if we where there, as we had been away so long. I think they thought we had done a bunk!

At some point I go to pharmacy to collect Water tablets and Potassium tablets, while Sue has a blood test. The pharmacist advises me to dissolve the potassium tablets in water and then add fresh orange juice to disguise the taste.

We eventually get home mid-afternoon, tired and hungry.

FRIDAY 28/4/2004

We go to the clinic to restart the Docetaxel chemo'. This will be the third session, but there has been a gap of four weeks since the last dose and I am concerned that not only will Sue get a sore mouth again, but the long break will have allowed the cancer to recover too much. Rather like not completing your antibiotic course or not getting all the roots out of a rampant weed. So its fingers crossed for my darling Susie. I think they had a be bit of a problem finding a good vein this time, Sue is beginning to suffer from all these chemo' and drip insertions.

In the evening we have a phone call from my sister saying my Dad has gone into hospital with a low heart pulse rate. They plan to do an operation to fit a pacemaker on the following Tuesday.

The in-laws have triumphed again, and stolen Sue's thunder!

SATURDAY 29/5/2004

Sue is high on the steroids and as we go up to see her Mum, on the way we end up arguing about the way I am driving her car!

Post card to Dad in hospital. First communication for some time, but Susie insists on me sending it; how right she was to be!

SUNDAY 30/5/2004

Dad leaves hospital, as apparently there is no way they can do the operation for a fortnight! Goes off with other sister. My card will not arrive now until after he has gone home!

MONDAY 31/5/2004

I am worried, my concern about Sue's mouth ulcers returning looks like happening.

WEDNESDAY 2/6/2004

Dash out to Argos and buy a V-pillow to help support Sue's head so she can sleep easier. She has been using about six pillows to support her, as she will not lie down for fear of starting to cough again.* Also she can not relax and go to sleep, because she is frightened of not waking up again. Hence she has had very little sleep at night for sometime.

   * Sue has had a cough since a bout of "flu" at Christmas.

THURSDAY 3/6/2004

Blood test for chemo' on Friday, drop Sue at entrance and then park car, as near possible to the entrance. Short wait for test as they are not very busy and we might get away with a free half hour. On leaving we discover car park ticket machine is not working and I have to run/walk round to the nearest one only to discover I am well over the time limit, so it costs £2.

   Mum rings to say she needs to go the dentist as soon as possible as she has a sore gum. Sue H. had agreed to take Sue to tomorrow's chemo' session and I was going to have a day off, now it looks like I shall have to take Mum if the dentist will fit her in.

FRIDAY 4/6/2004

Take Mum to dentist who prescribes antibiotics and pain killers and asks her to come back in a week.

   Sue and Sue H. off to clinic for chemo' at 1.00pm. They arrive home very late, as the nurses had terrible trouble finding a vein in Sue's arm/hand. Dr. E. has prescribed new water tablets and a different sort of potassium tablet (smaller), hopefully easier for Sue to swallow. They were so long on the vein hunt that they nearly gave up, before one of the doctors succeeded, just as Dr. E. was going to call it a day. So this is the last Docetaxel chemo' and she will now be put on a pill called Xeloda, which is the last paddle for Sue's canoe. Hope it works! I was surprised they had given Sue the Docetaxel, because her mouth was already becoming very sore, but as I wasn't there I didn't have a say! Pity!

TUESDAY 8/6/2004

Very worried about Sue, so I ring the hospital and spoke to Kate explaining Sue has got really bad mouth ulcers again. Kate advises me to ring the doctor tomorrow or the ward if I am not happy with Sue's condition. I know Sue should really be back in hospital but she wants to be at home, so I leave it until tomorrow.

'Sue is trumped again'. We have a phone call from my younger sister at 11.10pm, to say Dad has died sometime that evening, neighbours/ police found him. It was all quite peaceful they think. Dad had received our card; it had been re-directed by the hospital, thank goodness.

Oh dear what else can go wrong, first my Mum (last October), then an Aunt (February) and now Dad. Also a friend from the local Organ Association and a workmate both died in the same week in October last year!

WEDNESDAY 9/6/2004

Call local GP doctor to see Sue. Arrives in the late morning. I have to do a lot of the explanations as to all Sue's problems and the chemo' history, as she can not talk very well. He prescribes a liquid for Sue's sore mouth and morphine for the pain. I collect the items later and we start immediately on these medicines. The mouth medicine involves pouring a 1ml of a liquid on to a small spoon and then upturning it onto Sue's tongue, all without touching her mouth as it is very painful. Thank goodness I have a very steady hand, as it would be impossible otherwise.

Veronica calls round with a single Iris in a very nice tall jar for Sue, she doesn't stay. I thought it was Irene and Angela who phoned earlier saying they would call round in the evening to leave some flowers and a card as they will be off on holiday soon. When they come Sue is too tired and will not see them, I have a chat with them outside. They are very kind and we have hugs all round. Wish them luck on their holidays and they will phone early next week to see how Sue is getting on.

THURSDAY 10/6/2004

Sue is no better, but wants to hang on until Friday when she is due to see Dr. E. for a check-up prior to her next chemo'. Her legs are very red and one of the blisters is starting to leak so we arrange towels on the bed to help catch the water. I am persuaded to wait until tomorrow, maybe I should have insisted on taking her up or recalling the doctor, but I think I am getting so tired with the strain and I don't insist.

I do dash out to Argos again hoping to buy two fans, one for Sue and one for the conservatory. As usual they are out of stock, not surprising really as it has been rather hot recently. I choose another model which in fact is excellent.

Irene had suggested getting one the day before, but I had dismissed the idea as I thought Sue would not been interested in one. However I was wrong and she asked for one. Ironic in a way, because for a long time she had been cold all the time, even in the conservatory which was well into the upper twenties centigrade at times in the sun.

FRIDAY 11/6/2004

We are due at the clinic at 1pm and as Sue is so bad, I ring to check to find out if they are on time at the clinic, as I don't think she should wait around for a long time. They are on time, so say they!

Wrong! We have a long wait on arrival, as some crisis has arisen in the meantime.

Just getting there was interesting as I had to help Sue in and out of the car, because she had become so stiff with her swollen legs and the blisters had got worse. We had a heated discussion in the car on the way, about Sue going into the hospital ward to get better support and treatment than I could give her at home.

Dr. E. takes one look at Sue's legs and suggests she admits herself to the ward, but Sue wants to go home. The expert on blister bandaging is called for and it turns out to be Sarah, who sets to work while I am sent to collect more morphine as Sue might need more over the weekend. I find the usual pharmacy closed and have to use the main one downstairs; it's very small, stuffy and hot. Not much of a queue but I still wait quite a long time. When I get back to the clinic I am called aside and asked to try and persuade Sue to come in on Sunday.

Dr. E. had already said to me in the corridor as I left for the pharmacy, Sue should not be going home, but I said if Sue wants to go home today I would try and persuade her to come in on Sunday.

In the meantime they have arranged for the district nurse to call on Saturday and re-bandage Sue's legs.

Eventually we are reunited and prepare to leave, I get the car round to the front door and Sue is helped in by two nurses from the clinic. They are very kind and gentle trying desperately to talk Sue into coming in on Sunday.

Get home exhausted! How Sue feels I can only imagine.

She must have had a long think about it and decided, for my sake 'so she said', that she would go in on Sunday. My thoughts are, that if she gets back to the ward she can have intra-venous drips of liquids and medicines to stop the mouth ulcers and get better for the Xeloda chemo'. With hindsight I had just not realised how desperately ill Sue was at this stage.

Sue H. rings in the evening and agrees to come over on Saturday afternoon to have a talk with Sue and me.

SATURDAY 12/6/2004
Sue's legs very bad. The district nurse arrives early and takes lots of details for her records and the hospital tomorrow. She raids her entire supplies of bandages, pads and incontinence mats to do a wonderful job on Sue's legs. The blisters are larger and more numerous, at least we can dispose of the towels now. Sue H. visits us and we have a long chat about the situation, Sue confirms she will go into the hospital tomorrow.

My Mum's birthday!

SUNDAY 13/6/2004
Sue had a very bad night, I had to help her on the toilet, which was the first time I felt inadequate and found the situation difficult. Sue of course had spent years cleaning messy children's bottoms at school, all part of the day's work in a special school! (Blocked drains!)

I arranged to meet Sue H. at the hospital main entrance; she would find a wheel chair. All I had to do was get Sue up, give her pills etc. and get her into the car. Swollen feet and bandages meant she couldn't wear shoes or slippers, so I put polythene bags on her feet to stop them dripping on the carpets. Unfortunately they leaked a bit in the car, but the rubber mats saved the day.

Thank goodness it was Sunday and very quiet outside the main entrance, so we could park and unload Sue straight into the wheel chair. At least we are expected in the ward as I had rung earlier and checked they had a bed for Sue.

Sue was installed in the other main ward this time, a bit bigger and quieter as it was a Sunday. We waited for Dr. Several to arrive and Sue was processed into the system again. I had to do a lot of the talking as Sue had a very sore mouth again. Dr. Several had great difficulty finding suitable veins for blood samples and the cannula, but in the end he did a good job. The nurse had un-bandaged Sue's legs so the doctor could see them, the blisters were terrible by now and she had to put her feet on mats to catch the liquid from them. Eventually Sue was put on a drip and given a new antibiotic, painkillers etc. but some had to be by mouth.

I stayed until lunch time, then went home saying I hoped to come back in the evening with her slippers and the spoon for her mouth medicine that was useful for swallowing things. I got home and did lots of washing and jobs, had tea and then sat down for thirty minutes snooze. I awoke an hour later with a start, heart pumping fast and felt terrible. I tried to recover but could not gather the strength to drive to the hospital again. So I retired to bed early hoping to feel fine in the morning, when I was due to visit Sue with Sue H. in the morning and Veronica was going in the afternoon.

MONDAY 14/6/2004

The next day I just could not face the prospect of visiting Sue, knowing I would probably have to help with feeding etc. I just felt it was somebody else's turn. So Sue went on her own and I managed to get Veronica to call and collect a card for Sue and her slippers. That eased my conscience a bit, promising Sue H. I would go on Tuesday with her.

They were installing communications equipment for patients at each bedside (well on the wall above) while the patients were still on the ward. This not only meant a lot of drilling and banging on the walls in the next bay, but Sue and others had to be moved around. So Sue ended up back in the original bay she started in the first time she was on the ward, but by the window instead of by the entrance.

TUESDAY 15/6/2004

Sue H. collected me and we got to the ward and of course found Sue had been moved. Sue seems a lot better, out of bed and we had good time talking and trying to help with drinks, ice lollies etc. her legs are a lot better. We tried to help her with lunch, she had a bit of broccoli to please me, but she only chewed as she couldn't swallow it. We had a break

103

for coffee and stayed until 1pm leaving for home in good heart, as she seemed to be improving.

That evening while I was peeling the potatoes, a staff nurse rang to say Sue wanted to talk to me. My poor Sue was very confused and wanted me to call the police, as she said "she was being held against her will in the ward". I spent some time trying to calm her down, agreeing to ask Veronica to call her husband (an ex-policeman) this seemed to settle her. At one point we were disconnected because Sue tried to dial 999. Poor darling she was badly affected by all the drugs she was being given and very frightened. With hindsight, I think it was her way of asking me to let her come home, as she didn't want to die alone in hospital. This situation was similar to a story she told about her and Dad when he was very ill with cancer. Eventually Sue was given something to calm her down and she did sleep a bit, I believe.

UNHAPPINESS

I can not forgive myself for not going to see Sue immediately; my excuse is, it was after 7pm and I would only unsettle her if I went. I could not bring Sue home, as she needed to be in hospital to have the antibiotics and saline drip, which I thought was going to make her better. I still had no idea how ill Sue really was, because if I had known I would have spent much more time with her. I am afraid I was just too tired to think, I thought another couple of weeks and Sue will be home again.

WEDNESDAY 16/6/2004

Veronica saw Sue in the morning and they had a chat about the phone call and Sue was a lot calmer as a result. When I went in the afternoon it was not mentioned. She was out of bed and we did a bit of chatting all afternoon. They gave her one of her antibiotics via a drip, but it took so long as it was in parallel with the saline solution; so by the time they started the second lot I decided to have a break and go for supper in the canteen. I wasn't gone long and on my return Sue was holding the end of the delivery tube and the antibiotic was dripping on the floor. In my panic I completely forgot the simple way to stop the flow using the sliding tap. (Squeezes the tube closed) so more than necessary went on the floor and the rest went in the rubbish bin. Eventually I went home about 6.30pm, although Sue didn't want me to go.

GUILT

I had no real idea that poor Sue was so very ill and I was still working on the assumption she would have one or two weeks in hospital to get over the ulcers in the mouth. Followed hopefully by time in the hospice, so they could get her eating and drinking before coming home and starting the Xeloda chemo'. The hospice stay would have been difficult to get Sue to do, but I had asked Kate to let the hospital staff suggest it as the best way forward. I know Sue H. has already mentioned it some while back and Sue was much against it, as she thinks it's a place to die only, not a place to recuperate and get more help with eating and drinking, than is possible on the ward.

THURSDAY 17/6/2004

Go to see Sue with Sue H. and we are both taken aback when we find Sue in bed behind curtains half drawn, with no drip attached, so she must be relying on her own drinking ability which is not good. We are very concerned, so I ask if I can speak to a staff nurse about Sue's condition. After a long time 'Matron' Sue's "friend", is available and we go off to a quiet room.

I am told Sue tried to get up in the night and in doing so pulled out her cannula, and would not let them try and put it back. I am not surprised as it must have hurt her badly and there are precious few places to try again. So it's down to Sue to try and drink and eat as there will not be any more saline drips. She can have medicines by mouth and injections but she must eat, so we are asked to help if we are around at lunchtime.

I report this to Sue H. and we try to help Sue with drinking. Sue can not talk at all really and we find it very difficult to understand what she wants, I suggest an ice lollipop, but it must not be orange, the only ones they have on the ward. So I dash off to the shop to get a tri-flavour ice lollipop. Sue eats this very quickly, even through her mouth is very sore and it was cold. Sue tries to say something to us, but we don't understand and suggest she writes it down. The result is unreadable, but we think it says 'I love Malcolm'.

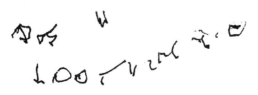

105

Everybody else seems to have had their lunch brought to them but not Sue, eventually it arrives, cold congealed mince and mashed potato, and not a chance a well person would attempt it, we tried Sue with a bit but she was not interested in food. Eventually she falls asleep and we go home at 1pm feeling relieved that she has at last managed to get to sleep and stay asleep.

At home I take some photographs in the garden and print them, to take up to Sue, something to show her and talk about tomorrow. She loves her garden and has spent many hours planting, weeding and propagating from cuttings.

I begin to wonder whether Sue is in a coma, not just sleeping, so I contact her Mum and say I will collect her and take her up to see Sue. We arrive around 4.30pm and Sue is still asleep, so things are not good for her, it really is a coma. I ring to tell Sue H. and she volunteers to come up but I say we will be okay.

I put Sue's Guardian Angel, Jennifer, in her left hand and she holds on to it tightly right to the end. Around 6pm we see Dr. E. and she is not sure whether its hours, days or weeks to the end.

We are offered lots of cups of tea, very British! Tea in a time of crisis! We wait in the relative's room while Sue is washed and tidied up and moved to the other bay, ironically back to the place she started in, which is more private as the room is larger. Sue's sister Mary is told and starts to dash over, a two and half hour drive to see Sue.

I try talking and reading to Sue from a magazine, to pass the time. I have a quick walk around the hospital grounds, luckily I was not long.

On my return Sue's breathing has become slower and I suddenly remember how she likes to be told a story, so I start to recount one of my stories about Pinkie the Elephant who goes for a walk to the seaside.

"Along the road down the hill to the bridge over the babbling brook, he stops to look at the water, then up the hill on other side from where he can see the sea down below with the waters of the brook flowing into the sea........."

Sue died at 9.25pm. Mary arrived too late.

My darling Susie I miss you very much, love Malcolm.

POSTSCRIPT

FRIDAY 18/6/2004

Visit the hospital to collect the death certificate. I find out I have to book an appointment at the registrar, to record the Sue's death, I manage to get one at 2.30pm. It's raining when we go, the first for weeks, I pay for three copies, as I know there will be plenty of people who will need to see it.

SATURDAY 19/6/2004

Mum and I visit the Undertakers and we organise details for the cremation. Mary, Sue's sister, is going on holiday so we hope we can get it arranged for Friday next week.

We go home and I spend a bit of time in the garden alone, as it's my father's funeral that morning in Inverness. No chance of going to it, even if I had wanted to go.

Later we drive to Newark to shop at Waitrose, a favourite place of us all, the meat is better than most other supermarkets, I think we had lunch as well.

SUNDAY 20/6/2004

The funeral will be on Friday at 11.10am. I start to think about the service for Sue, some organ music I think, but suddenly I can't remember any of the hymns she liked. We used to watch Songs of Praise together, a Sunday ritual, we had to make sure that supper was ready early, so as not to miss it and Sue often said "Oh I like that hymn".

MONDAY 21/6/2004

Start writing lists of all the people I must tell about Sue and arrange to see the solicitor next week, about the will.

TUESDAY 22/6/2004

Lots of people send sympathy cards, family and friends and her old colleagues from work.

THURSDAY 24/6/2004

Went to the funeral parlour to see Sue for the last time. On the way it started to rain, by the time I arrived it was pouring, with water gushing from the gutters and the roof. Good Omen?

Saw Sue on my own. Had a chat, but every time I tried to leave I couldn't. I just didn't want to leave her on her own. I shall miss her lots.

FRIDAY 25/6/2004

Funeral at the Lincoln Crematorium. Felt very calm. The weather was dry and sunny. The service went very well, the music I chose sounded okay. The Rev. E. conducted the service with dignity and said some nice things about Sue. Lots of Sue's friends from her old school came, some I knew, others I had met once or twice, others I knew by name only, a few of our neighbours and friends of mine also came.

• • • • • •

SUMMER 2004

I kept myself busy doing all the jobs we/I had started and not finished, the paving and steps outside the door to the conservatory, the gravel path around the remaining sides. Pruned shrubs, weeded flower beds, tidied up old piles of logs, sorted through all the plant pots Sue had filled with cuttings. She loved taking cuttings; most of them grew, so we were always looking for new places to put them. I managed to plant a few, such as Camellias, roses, Hydrangeas; the rest will have to await better weather in the spring now.

I miss Sue a great deal, as we had been a team for 24 years, thinking the same thoughts and doing things together. While I worked in the garden I could "forget" about Sue. I missed her greatly and often found little reminders of her would make me cry. I still find it difficult to believe she is not coming back, that I can't talk to her and tell all the latest news and gossip, that she and I will not be able to share all the new experiences of life together.

I found typing her book and my "diary bit" helped me understand her better and what she had been going through during her illness. As I had only read bits of it, in parts before, the early hopes and her very positive attitude towards the Chemo', Radiotherapy and Thyroid operation, contrast with the loss of morale and unhappiness that the cancer had returned so soon.

The pain she endured with those terrible mouth ulcers must have been unbearable. I just wish I had realised how ill she was and that she would not return home. I just feel so guilty that I did not spend more time at the hospital with her during those last few days, but I WAS CONVINCED SUE WOULD BE COMING HOME, after a week or two!

REMEMBRANCE
SATURDAY 4ᵀᴴ SEPTEMBER 2004

One of Sue's ambitions was to be part of the first team of ringers that rang a quarter peal on the newly augmented and re-hung bells at St Andrew's Church, Potterhanworth. Yvonne and family have been raising money, since the Millennium, for three new bells and a new frame for all six bells.

The bells were not ready until after Sue's death and as she had been part of the team who rang at Branston Church, where she rang the 4th, they very kindly agreed to dedicate the 4th bell at Potterhanwoth to Sue, when the new bells were blessed by Canon Raymond Rodger at a dedication service on the 4th September 2004.

THE FUNERAL OF
SUSAN SCOULLER

HELD AT THE LINCOLN CREMATORIUM ON FRIDAY 25th JUNE
2004 AT 11.10 AM

If I should go before the rest of you,
Break not a flower nor inscribe a stone;
Nor when I've gone speak in Sunday voice,
But be the usual selves that I have known.
Weep if you must ~ parting is hell,
But life goes on, so sing as well.
(Words attributed to Joyce Grenfell)

MUSIC

INTRO - Fantasy, BWV 572, in G by Johann Sebastian Bach

PSALM - No. 23 The Lord is my shepherd: therefore can I lack nothing.

HYMN - No. 397 Guide me, O thou great Redeemer

EXIT - Rhapsody No. 3 for Organ by Herbert Howells

A POEM

Remember

Remember happy days, those hazy lazy summer days.
The sun shines warm, the insects hum,
Time suspended, time for fun.

A stream to ford, to splash and paddle,
A conversation with the cattle.
Trees to climb, rooks a huddle,
A great big enormous puddle.

Remember brown autumnal days.
The wet look leaves,
Free fruit on trees,
Natures cycle of decay.

Remember winters icy slide,
How, on frosty nights I loved to hear
Ancient bells sound crisp and clear.

Remember sticky buds, catkins and brave
Bright flowers of spring.
Fledglings wobbling on the wing.

Will you remember all these to see?
Will you remember me?

(Sue Scouller)

Service taken by Rev Richard Eyre Team Rector, Hykeham Team
Ministry.
Funeral Directors Lincoln Co-operative Funeral Services.
DONATIONS TO THE MACMILLAN CANCER RELIEF.

• • • • • •

SUE

I've lost a friend,
A gentle friend,
A friend I hardly knew.
I hardly have the right to even miss her as I do.

I only met her four or five,
While cutting back mum's hedge,
I'm pretty sure she doubted on
The straightness of my edge.

We hit it off, quite slow at first,
We were some years apart.
But soon we caught each other's drift,
Like kids in secret art.

We chatted like a pair of foals,
We put the world to rights.
Eavesdroppers would have
Laughed at all the fancy of our flights.

The hedge was trimmed,
The lawn was cut.
The summer grew in green.
And Sue would ring reminding me,
To cut the lawn again.

I knew that she had fallen ill,
But didn't think to know,
The fullness of its course
Would mean that she would have to go.

I heard the church bells peal just now,
While talking to a tree.
And missed this lady that I knew,
That now I'll never see.

Life isn't fair.
It isn't just.
It doesn't think we care.
For if it did,
You'd still be here.
With all those thoughts to share.

By Paul Jones